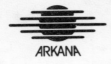

ARKANA

18/41.

How to Relieve Arthritis

Michael Blate is well known as a leading teacher and authority in the art (or science) of self-health. He has appeared on nationwide radio and television in Britain and the USA, and is the author of more than a dozen books in the field of natural health and healing without drugs or medicines, including *The Natural Healer's Acupressure Handbook: G-Jo Fingertip Technique*, *Advanced G-Jo*, *How to Heal Yourself Using Hand Acupressure*, *How to Heal Yourself Using Foot Acupressure*, and (with Gail Watson) *Cooking Naturally For Pleasure and Health*, all published by Routledge & Kegan Paul.

How to Relieve Arthritis

The Acugenic Method

Michael Blate
with Gail C. Watson, M.S.

ARKANA

London, Melbourne and Henley

First published in 1985
by ARKANA PAPERBACKS
ARKANA PAPERBACKS is an imprint of
Routledge & Kegan Paul plc

14 Leicester Square, London WC2H 7PH, England

464 St Kilda Road, Melbourne,
Victoria 3004, Australia and

Broadway House, Newtown Road,
Henley-on-Thames, Oxon RG9 1EN, England

Typeset by Columns, Reading
Printed and bound in Great Britain by
The Guernsey Press Co Ltd,
Guernsey, Channel Islands
Copyright © Michael Blate 1985

ISBN 1-85063-010-0

This book is dedicated to my mother, Sylvia Lax Blate, who has shown me through her silent courage the kind of suffering arthritis can bring.

Michael Blate

Contents

Contents

Important

If you are presently taking medication but have decided to try the G-Jo Institute 'all-natural' (drugless) way to self-treat arthritis, either in conjunction with, or as an alternative to total medical treatment, there are several steps it is wise to take first:

* Discuss this course of action with your doctor for his approval and suggestions . . .
* Unless otherwise suggested by your doctor, only withdraw from any regularly-taken medication (especially if taking cortisone or corticosteroids) *slowly and gradually* – especially if you have been under medication for a long time.

This book is presented as a catalog and primer of techniques and other information that have been in continuous use throughout the Oriental and Western world for many years. While these techniques and information utilize a natural system within the body, there are no claims made for their effectiveness, even when properly used. These techniques and information are not an alternative to proper medical care and treatment, nor are they intended to supersede or replace any standard, Western medical techniques.

What is the G-Jo Institute?

The G-Jo Institute is a not-for-profit natural health research and educational organization. It was informally organized in 1976 and incorporated in 1982. Its purpose is the dissemination of drugless 'self-health' techniques.

G-Jo is a simplified form of acupuncture without needles (or 'acupressure'). However, the scope of the G-Jo Institute has expanded far beyond its original purpose of the sharing of simple acupressure techniques.

It is our belief that it is the body-mind – and *only* the body-mind – which heals itself. For that reason, we now address ourselves to the *entire* spectrum of how to stimulate the innate self-healing mechanisms within the body-mind with simple, yet effective, self-applied techniques from around the world.

For further information or catalogs about our publications, recordings, workshops and such, send a business-sized, self-addressed stamped envelope (or equivalent international postage stamps for locations outside the U.S.A.) to:

THE G-JO INSTITUTE
DIVISION-AR
POST OFFICE BOX 8060
HOLLYWOOD, FLA. 33024
U.S.A

Acknowledgments

The authors gratefully wish to acknowledge Sandy Pasquale for her unceasing efforts and cooperation in the face of deadline after deadline.

We also wish to thank Andrea Holly Gold for her willingness to edit this manuscript at all hours of the day and night, and again to Andrea – and Laurie Sue Blate – for their enthusiastic preparations of the recipes herein for The G-Jo Institute's 'Taste-tested Stamp of Approval.'

What is ACUGENICS?

'Acugenics' means *that which has its basis in the acupuncture (energy) theory*. This traditionally-Oriental viewpoint believes that a vital force – called *bioenergy* – circulates from organ to organ throughout the body, making them produce the chemicals and electromagnetic impulses vital for life.

When bioenergy is moving smoothly from organ to organ – neither too quickly nor too slowly – we are in good health. But when any disruption or malfunction occurs within the energy system, symptoms appear and we are considered to be ill. In this Oriental point of view, there are thousands of symptoms but only one disease: an 'imbalanced' flow of bioenergy.

ACUGENICS is the program developed at The G-Jo Institute, based on this traditional Eastern way of healing; but it is expanded to also incorporate other easy, self-health methods, both from modern science as well as from the first-hand experiences of many individuals in self-treating their own ailments. ACUGENICS incorporates acupressure, medicinal diet, vitamins and many other drugless, easy-to-use methods for 'whole-person' healing and wellness.

Foreword

As a doctor reading this book about arthritis, I am immediately struck by its breadth of scope. For 'arthritis,' as we are taught in our medical training, is a disease affecting the joints and connective tissues of the body; literally, an inflammation of the joints. In dealing with arthritis we have been led to focus down on this specific aspect of the body and to gear our treatments solely to the relief of pain and inflammation in the joint areas.

We have been led to consider the problem in a manner similar to the way we would approach a malfunction in our automobile: namely, that the machine (in this case, the human body) has had some breakdown in its mechanical functioning. With that limited viewpoint, the solution is obvious: repair or replace the part; or – what is typically done in body-medicine – relieve as much suffering as possible, restore at least some modicum of function, and otherwise 'make do.'

In short, the doctor's advice for arthritis sufferers is typically a statement of the 'reality' that the patient will just have to 'live with it,' along with directions to take some prescribed medication that may make the job of living with it a little easier and less painful. Our doctors, in fact, tend to view our 'disease' as a kind of enemy that must be dealt with firmly for having had the audacity to have stepped into our lives in the first place.

There are millions of arthritis sufferers, and the medical journals are replete with drug advertisements promising the doctor that he, in turn, may promise his patients relief, with some hope of positive outcome. But in many – probably most – cases, the drugs have not given the patient a satisfying result. Worse yet, they have frequently produced side effects that have caused patients (like you!!) even more discomfort and suffering. Lately, the drug advertisers have been favoring a 'get tough' policy, touting new and more potent medications. I quote from just such an ad: 'Get tough with arthritis. Get tough with double-strength (name of product). Twice the strength of the original formulation.'

You have in your hands a tool that will not admonish you to 'get tough.' In fact, as you will see, it may be just that kind of attitude of dealing with things in your life that has aided your development of arthritis. And you will not be advised to take 'extra strength' pills, though you will be reminded of the INNER STRENGTH you may call upon to help you regain some power over your life and over your dis-ease.

You will be guided to adopt a viewpoint of looking at *all* of you – your whole body, mind, emotions, and spirit – as the 'patient' rather than picturing the problem as being just in your joints. And you will see that your attitudes and feelings, the foods you eat, the way you breathe, and the environment you live in (including the company you keep) all play a part in creating your illness. In seeing this you will gain some new perspectives on how to REVERSE your dis-ease, so as to create the feeling of comfort, health, and mobility that you desire.

This is a book that truly offers a wider perspective on the subject of arthritis. It will help you see that the key to feeling good is to mobilize your will to heal yourself and then to realize how much you *can* do to help yourself, your family, and your friends. There are many doctors who have adopted this point of view and many others joining the ranks of those who would choose to help you help yourself rather than have you be the passive recipient of the latest armamentarium of drug treatments.

Britain's Prince Charles is one such notable personality: in his address before the British Medical Association at its 150th anniversary, he urged doctors to use more natural methods of healing whenever possible; and to work more in collaboration with patients rather than treating them as broken-down machines in need of repair. He made reference to the high cost, both in terms of money and discomfort (morbidity) of our drug-oriented methods of cure. Said the Prince, 'I would suggest that the whole imposing edifice of modern medicine, for all its breathtaking successes is, like the celebrated Tower of Pisa, slightly off balance.'

I wish you success in using this book as a way of balancing some of the excesses that may have played a part in your development of arthritis. And I hope that you may experience some of the pure pleasure that comes from having your own Tower of Pisa back on firm footing again. The choice is yours.

Barry Sultanoff, M.D.
Medical Director,
The G-Jo Institute,
Davie, Florida

Introduction

We in the West have grown up with the erroneous, but wide-spread idea that, should disease (or 'dis-ease') strike, there is little we can actually do on our own to treat it (beyond reaching for the aspirin or other over-the-counter medication). 'New' ideas (such as some of those presented in this work) are greeted with great skepticism. The feeling is that, if the remedy is so good, why aren't doctors using it ... or at least why haven't we heard of it before?

In the East, where doctors are few and poverty is much more common than in Western Europe or America, people have long realized that there is an *enormous* amount that one can do for him- or herself. In fact, many centuries ago Orientals realized that disease does not generally strike without many advance warnings; they also recognized that dis-ease arose from 'insults' or abuse to the system. Having realized this, they deduced that by stopping the abuse, the body could self-heal. For even thousands of years ago, these wise people observed that it is the body – and *only* the body – which heals itself.

However, it was also learned that there were ways to *stimulate* self-healing. Some of these methods were 'physical' (such as acupressure or exercise – both of which are covered in this program), mental (such as meditation or 'visualization') ... and some were even spiritual (prayer, for example).

Furthermore, not only did they learn that there are at least several remedies for most diseases (even serious ailments), but in most cases there may actually be *dozens* of techniques and methods which can stimulate self-healing. It is my purpose, and the purpose of The G-Jo Institute, to share some of the less foreign and more-easily accomplished of these methods I have been introduced to in my travels and studies.

It is important to realize that the remedy, itself, does not cause healing; at best, it can only stimulate the body to do its normal job of restoring health (or, as the Orientals would say, 'restoring balance') within itself. Thus it would not be expected to use *all* the remedies and methods described in the following pages. Sometimes using even just a few methods – perhaps doing nothing more than simply *desiring* to become (or to suddenly have a reason to be) healed is all that it takes for dramatic results to occur.

Admittedly, this is unusual . . . but not unheard of. On a more practical basis, however, you are advised to immediately put into use any and all of those methods which cause you little or no inconvenience, and especially those which 'feel right' to you intuitively. As you begin feeling better, then perhaps add more of the methods which require larger changes in your daily life. Your sincere desire to rid yourself of your suffering is the key to self-healing: the remedies only accelerate the process. But they do this powerfully well – even the most apparently simple techniques described herein.

So it is with great pleasure I now present to you a veritable catalog of 'people-proven' remedies and methods; and I urge you to select generously from this menu . . . you will not be disappointed! To the extent you seriously use these techniques, to that same extent you should enjoy relief from your suffering.

On a final note, I strongly suggest that no matter what other of the methods or techniques you incorporate, that the first and foremost of these be the use of acupressure (acupuncture without needles – see the final pages of Section III). In nearly every case, the results will be nothing short of astounding. I have not included such techniques as acupuncture or homeopathy, two extremely powerful and effective (yet normally safe and gentle) methods, only because they are not generally self-applied. But I strongly urge you to seriously investigate one or both of these methods, to use in conjunction with this ACUGENICS program.

Good luck . . . and best wishes for health and wellness!

Michael Blate
Executive Director
The G-Jo Institute

A Note to Readers

Before starting this program, it is important for you to think about – and accept – several important facts about your arthritis:

1. Something – and often many things – in your lifestyle is unhealthy and is contributing to your illness.

2. You are ill and suffering, not just from a physical ailment called 'arthritis,' but from emotional and spiritual distress, as well. Arthritis is a 'whole-person' dis-*ease*.

3. To become well and 'reverse' (heal) your dis-ease as much as possible, you must first WANT to get well . . . the intention and desire to heal yourself is as important as any therapy or technique. Without that intention to get well, you can never restore and enjoy health and well-being!

4. While many of these techniques are surprisingly easy, all of them have helped others find relief from, and often 'reversal' (healing or long-term relief) of, arthritis; but you must allow yourself enough time for the techniques to show these effects . . . and while you may notice some benefits almost immediately, solid results could take a month or longer to appear.

5. You should prepare yourself for a certain amount of initial inconvenience as well as for a long-term – even

a life-long – commitment to the principles and techniques described in this program. In any event, you should expect your life to change – often substantially – but invariably for the better as you follow this program.

6. Various types of arthritis are possible symptoms of such problems as worms (or similar intestinal parasites), certain vitamin deficiencies (esp. vitamin C, P, D, B_5 and/or B_6), certain mineral deficiencies (e.g. sodium, iodine, magnesium, hydrogen and/or sulphur) or even gradual, long-term poisoning by various pollutants (such as lead, arsenic or aluminum). For this reason, it is always wise to first have a complete medical check-up – including such non-traditional tests as hair analysis or cytotoxic testing (for hidden food allergies) – before beginning any form of self-treatment. (Note: when such poisoning is present, it may usually be easily purged with various homeopathic remedies – check with your homeopathic physician.)

7. Improving your own health is *always* a trade-off: you give up or release an abuse (such as smoking) with the expectation of a benefit (living longer, feeling better, etc., in exchange for the 'pleasure' that smoking brought). What are the benefits for the trade-offs in *this* program? In return for your patience, efforts and commitment, you should expect to receive an immediate sense of relief from pain . . . a more relaxed and 'emotionally-centered' state of being . . . a greater sense of optimism . . . a less restricted feeling of love for yourself, your family and friends, your world . . . and a growing sense of spiritual upliftment.

Section I:
Understanding your Arthritis

Arthritis – the crippler that affects women five times more frequently than men – seems to be caused by a combination of imbalanced or incomplete nutrition, in combination with a hereditary predisposition to this type of suffering; and nearly always, arthritis sufferers have feelings of harsh, unresolved and unvented emotional distress.

Arthritis has been called 'The Resentment Disease,' 'The Hidden Anger Disease,' 'The Woman's Crippler,' among other names. While it is primarily painful inflammation of the joints, it may affect bones, ligaments, tendons and organs, as well. Arthritic symptoms usually begin manifesting themselves before the age of forty.

It is primarily a chronic joint disability which includes nearly 100 different symptoms. 'Arthritis' is actually a catchall or umbrella term that includes *gout, osteoarthritis, rheumatoid arthritis, bursitis, rheumatism, menopausal arthritis,* etc.

Arthritis has been treated medically by numerous substances; and while some medical therapies have been temporarily effective, most have proven themselves eventually useless or even harmful. Several common medications are frequently used to relieve arthritis – aspirin, gold, cortisone and 'The Pill' (oral contraceptive) – all of which have potentially harmful side-effects.

Arthritis is often associated with excessively low blood pH (blood that is too acid). Certain 'extreme' foods (explained below) – especially those which create or perpetuate this state of blood hyperacidity – appear to 'leach out' vital nutrients from the system (an important way by which the body's chemical balance is disrupted), so you must avoid those foods as much as possible (details below).

However, proper eating is not enough to completely reverse or heal arthritis, because it did not begin with (but *is* greatly aggravated by) 'wrong' food. Arthritis appears to be rooted in the *emotions* – or even deeper, in spiritual distress (if the traditional Oriental viewpoint is correct). So for the best results of this program, you'll have to use other self-applied therapies – especially methods which help you to deal at least with the emotions (as well as the pain and physical suffering of arthritis) in conjunction with any dietary tactics.

There are ten important categories in The G-Jo Institute's arthritis ACUGENICS program. The basis of this program originated in the Orient and has been in use for thousands of years. It is an application of the so-called 'energy theory' of healing and wellness – the same theory that is the basis of acupuncture and other forms of 'energy medicine.' The information in each category plays a vital part in creating a whole-person or *holistic* approach for relieving and healing yourself. Please read this entire program before beginning any techniques or methods described herein. The ten categories include the following:

1. Good preventive and/or therapeutic foods (to be added to your diet);
2. Common excesses, abuses or irritants (to be avoided);
3. Preventive and/or therapeutic vitamins;

4. Preventive and/or therapeutic minerals and other supplements;
5. Other common needs and deficiencies of arthritis sufferers (to be added to your 'healthstyle');
6. Important 'external' therapies (e.g. exercise, etc.);
7. Preventive and/or other therapeutic herbs or other 'natural medicines';
8. Meditation-type techniques plus specific prayers and visualizations (to promote subconscious change and spiritual upliftment);
9. Important 'acupressure' (acupuncture without needles) methods and techniques – the key to the success of ACUGENICS;
10. Delicious recipes using many of the 'arthritis-fighting' foods described in Category One.

As implied earlier, an illness cannot be divided between body and mind, for body and mind are actually one. In this program, it is assumed that our 'mind' extends from the body's various organs and glands, and is 'manipulated' by the electro-magnetic energy and the biochemicals these organs and glands produce.

In other words, when we change our 'electro-chemical' balance (produced by the organs and glands in action), we change how we feel both physically *and* emotionally. This is how drugs and medicines work – and this is how *this* program works, as well.

This is because it is the body-mind – and *only* the body-mind – which heals itself. Drugs, medications or even the methods in this program are only assistants to the natural process of self-healing.

Furthermore, according to many holistically-oriented healers, the 'body-mind' is only a manifestation of the spiritual part of the human being – the part sometimes called the 'soul.' Thus, the body-mind is subsequent to the spirit-soul . . . the spirit's servant, as it were. Ultimately, it is said that *all* disease represents first a spiritual disorder within the sufferer.

Consequently, no complete healing is possible unless and until *spiritual* well-being is restored. In this regard, most Western as well as Eastern natural health authorities agree that some kind of spiritual practice greatly aids the process of healing. This may be in the form of prayer, humane service to another person or group, regularly studying Holy Scriptures, etc.

There are at least 12 major organs and glands within your body. These include: the lungs; colon; stomach; spleen-pancreas; heart; small intestine; urinary bladder; kidneys; nervous system; digestive (including endocrine) glands; gallbladder; and liver.

Each of them directly or indirectly controls one or more mental/emotional functions, according to the Oriental doctor-philosophers who discovered and developed the energy (acupuncture) theory of health – the basis of this program.

When our electro-chemical mixture is too 'rich' in one substance – say, insulin (a product of the digestive glands, stimulated by the liver interacting with the spleen, pancreas and other organs) – predictable emotional responses nearly always occur (e.g., anger, depression and/or hostility). Knowing this, it becomes easier to understand why sugar – which triggers an excess flow of insulin – is one of the foods that will be suggested arthritis sufferers avoid. This common 'food' tends to create not only anger and its subsequent reaction, depression, but also to increase one's sensitivity to pain. This is because the liver – which is greatly affected by sugar – is also the primary organ 'in charge of' regulating the level of pain one feels.

Furthermore, an excess of one or more such biochemicals must also produce a deficiency in others. Thus, the effects of electro-chemical imbalance within our system are two-sided – excessive in some areas, deficient in others – and create many complicated problems. Arthritis, a many-faceted dysfunction, is just one of them.

Until better balance is restored, health problems will continue to plague us. This is especially true of arthritis (because it is such a complex problem).

Each food, thought and activity we experience is believed to have an immediate effect upon our electro-chemical balance. So the goal of this natural self-health program is *to teach you* simple methods *to help restore internal harmony* – and to maintain it as completely as possible – through easy, regular practices and avoidances. When this vital balance is restored, your arthritis will – *must* – diminish and be relieved.

The Emotions Which are Connected to Arthritis

Arthritis is best characterized by *emotional inflexibility* or a *low 'adaptability factor.'* In other words, arthritis sufferers tend to be rigid and fixed in their views of the world. The stronger the opinions held, the greater their suffering tends to be.

Arthritis sufferers often hold strong 'romantic' illusions – such as fairy tale notions or impossibly high ideals – about what life 'should be.' At the core of this fantasy is usually found the sufferer's attitude about male-female relationships – especially his or her own.

At least in a female sufferer's case, this attitude is nearly always one of *resentment*. The greater a woman resents her (real or imagined) role as a female and mate, the greater her potential of suffering from arthritis. Male arthritis sufferers often carry hidden anger and resentment directed towards employers or superiors in business or work.

Rheumatoid arthritis is often suffered by someone who hides resentment and hostility by 'putting on a good face.' Osteoarthritis sufferers are often unusually *fearful*, as well as resentful. Gout – which is generally triggered by a rich, fatty diet (and which tends to affect males more frequently than females) – may be rooted in hidden fears of *deprivation* and *starvation* (a common emotional symptom of obesity, too). Other forms of arthritis have their own special emotional wellsprings, as well.

While it is possible to intellectually understand that these emotions may exist within ourselves, becoming *fully* aware of their influence is far more difficult. The pain and suffering from arthritis may actually be serving the purpose of *protecting* us from the pain of having to directly confront those hard-to-handle feelings. But until we recognize that our unvented emotions and feelings are the roots of this illness, we can usually expect only temporary relief from suffering.

Though arthritis affects the entire body-mind, there are three major organs which are primarily responsible for most arthritic suffering: the lungs, the kidneys and the liver. Only by restoring especially these organs to a better state of balance and functioning can arthritis actually be reversed.

Left unchecked and uncontrolled, however, the arthritic man or woman may also expect to suffer from at least several other common, related symptoms:

* gallbladder problems;
* dry skin, dry mucous membranes;
* low or erratic blood pressure;
* bronchitis and night cough;
* deformed hands, feet;
* wry neck;
* anemia;

* craving for acids, acidic foods;
* colitis;
* constipation;
* acute allergic reactions;
* nearly constant pain;
* cataracts or other eye disorders;
* edema, especially in the ankles;
* emotional distress;
* painful toes and fingers;
* bone spurs;
* tendency to form kidney stones;
* frequent leg cramps;
* joint stiffness;
* arteriosclerosis, etc.

As you see, whatever small inconvenience may be experienced by changing diet and 'healthstyle' will be compensated by reducing – perhaps completely avoiding – the above symptoms (most of which will be *very* inconvenient and unpleasant).

Section II:
Nutritional Remedies and Data

Foods Which Often Help Relieve and Reverse Arthritis

There are over 100 foods, supplements, techniques and methods described in the following pages which have been successfully used to control and help reverse arthritic suffering. In the beginning of this program, it is wise to first select or try any foods, vitamins, minerals, herbs or methods that intuitively 'feel right,' 'seem good,' or 'sound tasty' to you.

You already have a subtle knowledge of what *is* right for you; and allowing this 'intuitive guidance' ability to 'bloom' will be a most important tool in the on-going job of healing yourself.

The foods below are known as 'arthritis-fighters' because of their ultimate effects on pain, inflammation and other symptoms of arthritis. Use several – even many (in moderation!) – for it doesn't matter *what* remedies work for you, only that they help to bring relief and stimulate self-healing. The recipes in the final section of this book are based around many of these foods (the most important of these foods are *underlined*).

* grapefruit (including the white membrane);
* pumpkin seeds;
* raw goat's milk;

* yogurt (esp. from goat's milk);
* green, leafy vegetables;
* buttermilk;
* red beets;
* <u>strawberries</u>;
* wheat grass (sprouted wheat seeds);
* sour apples;
* kelp and other sea vegetables;
* watercress;
* millet;
* potatoes (juice of <u>raw</u> potatoes – please note: potatoes are an 'extreme' food and may as easily aggravate an arthritic condition as relieve it; this is especially true for any kind of <u>fried</u> potatoes – use trial and error testing);
* brown rice;
* yams;
* celery;
* sesame seeds or tahini;
* parsley (in moderation);
* sunflower seeds;
* garbanzo beans;
* wheat bran;
* sauerkraut (but watch the salt);
* tofu (bean curd);
* rice bran;
* agar-agar;
* pectin (e.g. 'Certo');
* asparagus;
* parsnips;
* broccoli;
* squash;
* rutabagas;
* lettuce;
* peas;
* chard;

* carrots;
* cauliflower;
* endive;
* oatmeal;
* sour cherries;
* bananas;
* pineapple;
* wheat germ;
* most beans (dried, not canned, if possible);
* avocados;
* pecans;
* fresh tomato juice (note: this is another 'extreme' food – like potatoes – so avoid it if you notice it causes any distress);
* alfalfa, especially sprouted;
* turnips;
* most bean sprouts;
* string beans;
* cold-pressed oil (esp. peanut and/or olive).

In the final pages of this book are found numerous delicious, easy-to-fix recipes for using many of these foods. Each of these meals has been 'people-tested' and enthusiastically endorsed by members of The G-Jo Institute.

The best 'arthritis-fighting' diet appears to be a vegetarian diet, with the main emphasis being upon whole grains (especially brown rice) plus fresh fruits, nuts and vegetables grown within 50 miles of home. In other words, it is wise to eat *regionally and seasonally* whenever possible. It is important to remember that *food itself does not cure; it only stimulates the body-mind, through the organs and glands, to heal itself.*

For this reason, moderation is extremely important in taking *any* food and drink. Even the 'best' foods taken in excess can create chaos in the body-mind.

The way we eat is important, too: chewing for a long time – because of its effect on the liver, a main organ for controlling one's sensitivity to pain – is almost as beneficially important as the food itself. As a goal to strive for, *chew small bites of 'right' foods for a long time (up to 100 times).*

Ideally, a 'vegan' – or even a fruitarian (fruit and nuts only) – diet appears to be the most natural and (in a *low-stress environment*) also the most healthful. The vegan diet consists of *no* animal products, whatsoever (not even milk, cheese, other dairy products or eggs).

However, as a practical alternative for providing a 'completely' balanced diet (for most high-stress Western lives), a 'lacto-vegetarian' diet (see below) is probably best. This type of diet suggests using a small amount of milk, cheese (make sure it is *rennetless*, or hardened with *vegetable* – not glandular – rennet, available at most health food stores . . . at least in America), along with other dairy products, except eggs.

Any meat or slaughtered product appears to be unhealthy because, when a creature is slaughtered, its terror chemicals infect the meat. Aside from slaughtered food being both unnecessary for human health and inhumane, the end product of the slaughtered creature's terror – in the form of harsh hormones and biochemicals – finds its way into the ultimate consumer. Because of its effects on the kidneys and adrenals, this animal protein creates and fuels a high level of stress, fear and muscular tension within the consumer – states of being which an arthritis sufferer is most wise to avoid.

The G-Jo Institute 'Basic' Diet

There is a 'basic' diet – based on the lacto-vegetarian way of eating – which may be used by virtually everyone

11

without fear of nutritional deficiency. It may be adjusted downwards (for weight loss) or upwards (to maintain or increase weight) as necessary, and has essentially been approved by most leading Western health agencies (including The American Medical Association).

This diet is based on a 'numbers-of-servings-per-day' arrangement. There are four basic groups which include:

* The milk group – include at least *two* servings each day of the following foods: one cup of whole, low-fat or skim milk; one cup of buttermilk; one cup of low-fat yogurt; one cup of dry or low-fat cottage cheese; two slices of (preferably) rennet-less cheese.

* The protein group – include at least *two* servings daily of the following foods: one cup (cooked) dried beans; one cup dried peas; one cup dried lentils; one half to three quarters cup of (unsalted) nuts or peanuts; one cup of soybeans or soybean products (e.g. tofu, bean curd, tempeh, etc.); (optional, but not recommended – two eggs);

* The grain/cereal group – include at least *four* servings daily of the following foods (selecting whole grain or unrefined products whenever possible): one slice of bread; one roll, bun or muffin; one half to three quarters cup cooked or ready-to-eat cereal; one half to three quarters cup of rice; one half to three quarters cup of pasta (macaroni, noodles, spaghetti);

* The fruit/vegetable group – include at least *four* servings daily of any fresh fruit or vegetable (in moderate amounts), which may be taken either in whole or juice form. (Note: when taking fruit or vegetable juice, please remember to either *dilute* or take only a *small* – not a large – glass of

the whole juice. One 'normal' glass of, say, apple juice may have the equivalent of as many as *five* apples in it!).

These foods should ideally be consumed in five or six smaller meals throughout the day, rather than two or three larger meals – especially if weight loss is the goal. Largest meals should be consumed earlier in the day with only light snacking (of healthful foods from the above groups) occurring later in the day or evening.

This diet will generally provide enough vitamins, minerals, protein, calories and other nutritional requirements for a person leading a moderately-active-to-active lifestyle. For the average person trying to lose weight, 1200 to 1600 calories a day from the above food selections should provide a gradual and sustainable weight loss. Over 1600 calories a day will generally either maintain or increase weight, depending on your job, stress level, etc.

It is wise, however, to reduce – then eliminate – all dairy products (milk, cheese, etc.) as quickly as possible. These foods are a major source of 'hidden' allergic reactions (see information below). Their primary benefit is simply to provide a non-slaughtered source of vitamin B$_{12}$ for 'beginning' vegetarians.

As mentioned earlier, the 'ultimate' diet – which might take many years of training to 'achieve' – is the fruitarian way of eating (fruits, nuts and other foods that 'fall into our hands' when the time for eating them is ripe). But this requires a low-stress environment plus, in most cases, a spiritual pathway or belief that supports this way of eating.

Aside from the recipes included in this book, arthritis sufferers should have at least one meal daily consisting of only raw vegetables, either whole or in the form of diluted, fresh juice.

An interesting way to serve raw vegetables – even if you hate raw food – is as a 'blended salad.' The best way to prepare a blended salad is to use a food processor (or perhaps a blender) and simply chop any fresh, local vegetables for a few moments, until some juice is seen on the bottom of the processor. Add a few drops of fresh lemon juice and cayenne (red pepper) for 'snap' and enjoy! Raw horseradish, too, can be a healthful addition. But please avoid salt – or, if you must use it, try a sea salt/vegetable combination available from your local natural-food or health-food store.

Your cooked vegetables should generally be lightly *steamed*, rather than fried, boiled or baked, etc. Steamed foods benefit the liver most, the organ which, as mentioned, is primarily responsible for controlling our tolerance or sensitivity to pain.

A 'hyperactive' liver – which often reveals its condition through *anger, hostility, inward-turned aggressive emotions, loud voice, flatulence, bowel disorders, frequent cursing (either verbalized or silently, in your own mind)*, etc. – practically guarantees that you will suffer more pain than someone whose liver is functioning more normally. (A further description of hyperactive and underactive organs – plus a discussion of their symptoms and methods of treatment – is found in Michael Blate's ADVANCED G-JO, available from this publisher).

Raw fruit juices, too, are recommended – in moderation. It is wise to use these as replacements for coffee, soft drinks (especially colas), tea, chocolate-based or alcoholic beverages. Nearly any raw fruit or vegetable juice – except raw *cabbage* and sweet citrus, such as *orange* or *tangerine* (each of which should generally be avoided) – has at least neutral and usually beneficial qualities. But caffeinated or sugary beverages have quite the reverse effect; they ultimately magnify pain and suffering.

However, even the 'best' and most healthy diet may contain foods or substances to which a hidden allergy exists (more completely covered in next segment of the text). This kind of reaction is called 'hidden' because, instead of the typical allergic reactions (e.g., coughing, sneezing, etc.), symptoms such as obesity, heart dysfunction or even arthritis are the manifestations.

How does one discover such hidden allergies? There are several self-test methods described below. But any food (even one of the above-recommended foods) which is consumed to excess – or which you find yourself often craving – is highly suspect.

Common Excesses, Abuses or Irritants That Trigger Arthritic Symptoms

There are a number of foods and other irritants that arthritis sufferers are wise to avoid as much as possible. The most important dietary avoidances include:

* sugar or sugary foods and drinks;
* eggs;
* slaughtered animal products, including organ meats, chicken, turkey or other poultry, cold cuts or any other meat products;
* all slaughtered seafoods, especially herring, anchovies, sardines and shellfish;
* paprika;
* salt;
* red or green bell peppers;
* tobacco;
* alcoholic beverages;
* 'recreational' drugs (e.g., marijuana, etc.);
* iron supplements;
* potatoes (esp. fried or french-fried);

* sweet citrus fruits;
* caffeine-rich foods or beverages (esp. chocolate, coffee, tea and colas);
* white bread, other refined wheat products (e.g. macaroni, spaghetti, etc.);
* eggplant;
* most dairy products (to excess – esp. milk, ice cream, whipped cream and any pasteurized product).

Since the above list includes many of the staples of today's 'normal' Western diet, it is not difficult to understand why arthritis is such a widespread disorder.

This is not to say that, in moderation, these foods necessarily *cause* arthritis in a perfectly healthy person – but they at least trigger emotional and physical suffering by throwing the body-mind into electro-chemical imbalance. When this occurs for a long enough period of time – months or years, perhaps – then negative emotions become fixed, perceptions are altered and viewpoints become increasingly rigid and restricted. And when combined with a hereditary or personality predisposition to arthritis, these foods and substances do indeed cause or aggravate existing arthritic symptoms, according to traditional Oriental doctors and healers.

Besides abusive foods and drinks, there are a number of other excesses, health disorders and abuses which appear to be intimately connected to arthritis and its suffering:

* smoking (especially harmful to women);
* malnutrition – even many overweight people suffer from malnutrition;
* physical stress;
* emotional tension;
* 'hidden' food allergies;
* injuries and other physical traumas (the subsequently healed areas often become arthritic in a

person prone to this disorder);
* cold, damp climates;
* drinking (anything) with meals;
* obesity (being more than 10% above ideal body weight);
* alkalosis – being too alkaline in the *stomach* (not the blood); usually caused by too many acidic foods, such as sugar.

This list does not necessarily include all the causes, excesses or abuses which trigger arthritis and the emotions that seem to lead to it in people who are so predisposed. But nearly all of the above are arthritis-linked abuses that can be curtailed, eliminated or released from our 'healthstyle' without great difficulty.

Hidden food allergies, however, are another problem. Everyone has them – and often these allergies exist to important staples in our diets which do not appear on the list of 'wrong' foods.

As a rule of thumb, generally those foods which we crave and would miss the most are the most highly suspect. And any food taken to excess has the possibility of causing an 'addiction' (which is akin to at least a temporary food allergy).

However, there are several self-applied methods for more clearly revealing our most likely allergens. They include: pulse testing; patch testing; and keeping a daily journal/diary (or similar record-keeping method) of our foods, moods and observations. They are best used together.

The Pulse Test

For this test, all you need is a watch with a sweep second hand (or some method for counting seconds) and a little time for self-testing. The technique is simple enough: first, determine your normal 'resting' pulse rate (the rate

17

just after awakening and before you put *anything* in your mouth – including a cigarette or toothpaste – and is best calculated by averaging that rate for several mornings in a row). Then eat a regular meal.

Record each food and beverage this meal contained (a good place to record that information is in your daily journal/diary – see below). Include any inhalant (e.g., cigarette tobacco, etc.) that preceded and/or followed it, too. Then take your pulse for one minute in each fifteen-minute period that follows the meal for the next hour and a half.

But rest for a few minutes before you take it. For proper testing, this should be done after each meal you eat during the test period of a week or two.

When you've eaten a meal that triggered a pulse jump of five percent or more, then do the patch test, as described below. Use a little of each substance that meal contained. Mark each patch carefully so that there won't be any confusion when you check the results. (Note: if the problem is in the additives or hidden ingredients that food contained, you'll only be able to identify the allergen as to brand.)

A more complete method of pulse testing – along with an in-depth explanation of allergies and their many disguises – is found in THE PULSE TEST by Arthur F. Coca, M.D. (Arc Books, Arco Publishing Co., New York).

The Patch Test

Here, you take a bit of each food (or just the suspected allergen) and place it on your inner forearm. Cover it with a small piece of gauze and tape it firmly in place for a day or so. Keep it dry. When you peel it off, if the skin in direct contact with the test product is reddened or shows any kind of reaction, you're probably allergic to that substance.

But the patch test isn't foolproof – you may not react to all your allergens with reddened skin, or you may mistake a tiny reaction for something else (and even allergens that cause only tiny reactions may have powerful effects on your health). You may even overlook it completely. And some allergens – like dust, dry heat or sunlight – can't be easily tested. Still, this simple test can reveal the vast majority of hidden food allergens in an easy, painless way.

The Journal/Diary

One of the easiest yet most effective 'self-psychotherapy' techniques is the simple act of writing down thoughts. This is a *powerful* method of catharsis and revealing hidden or subconscious emotions. Its value is dramatically increased when you also make this an ongoing health record by recording each food, drink or drug (medicinal or 'recreational' – e.g., tobacco, alcohol, etc.) that you consume.

The reason for this is both simple and practical. In an abused body – that is, in the organs and glands of a person who has not 'cleansed' himself through a vegetarian or fruitarian diet or through a prolonged fast – it may take as long as several days for a food's effects to manifest themselves both physically and emotionally. And since most people can't even remember what they had for yesterday's lunch, the only dependable method for identifying a 'trigger food' is to record everything you eat and then watch the patterns start appearing . . . which they surely will!

Preventive and/or Therapeutic Vitamins

Arthritis apparently creates/is created by *deficiencies* as

19

well as by excesses and other abuses. One of the most important of these deficiencies is a lack of certain vitamins.

Vitamins appear to be created within the organs themselves; they do not need to be derived (in fact, it is possible they *cannot* be extracted) from food. A particular nutritional supplement (or, for that matter, food) appears to *stimulate* the organs to produce a specific nutrient in a very complex and even miraculous process.

But this vital 'organ-response stimulation' can occur from other non-food sources as well. Sunshine, for instance, stimulates the production of vitamin D (ergosterol) when it irradiates the skin. And vitamin B_{12} – the vitamin that strict vegetarians try to find in sources other than animal products – apparently may be stimulated in some unusual ways such as walking barefoot for as little as 10 minutes a day in grass which still holds early morning dew! (It reputedly works by stimulating acupuncture points in the foot that 'control' the colon and liver, the organs 'in charge of' vitamin B_{12} in the body.)

In any event, vegetarians and even fruitarians (those who eat only tree- or vine-ripened fruit and nuts) have lived – and continue to live – long and healthy lives without outside sources of B_{12}... as long as stress is kept to a minimum.

Nutritional deficiencies may be temporarily remedied by taking oral supplements to stimulate the production of the body's own vitamins (as well as minerals and other nutritional needs, described in the next category). But this can be a complicated process (to do it correctly), since each vitamin requires certain other catalysts to do the job right. So a certain amount of intelligent study is needed to use vitamin pills properly.

However, even with intelligent forethought vitamin pills should be taken only for a limited amount of time – a maximum of a year (and preferably less) – and used in conjunction with the other methods described in this program. *There is no single path to reversing arthritis – it must be a holistic effort.*

Before beginning vitamin (or mineral) supplement self-treatment, it is wise to first make sure a need exists. There are now inexpensive, painless tests (e.g., hair analysis) which can quickly detect or confirm a vitamin (or mineral) deficiency. These, however, must usually be administered by (or at least sponsored by) a doctor or other health care professional.

The following vitamins have proven themselves useful in self-treatment of arthritis:

* vitamin A;
* vitamin B complex;
* additional B_2 (riboflavin);
* additional B_3 (niacin);
* additional B_5 (pantothenic acid);
* additional B_6 (pyridoxine);
* additional B_{12} (cobalamin);
* vitamin C – larger-than-normal doses initially (up to *five grams* daily – esp. for osteoarthritis);
* vitamin D;
* vitamin E (esp. for osteoarthritis);
* vitamin P (bioflavinoids).

Since each person is unique, it is difficult to suggest ideal amounts of each vitamin to take. A good suggestion is to begin by taking slightly more than is recommended on the bottle for several days, then reducing it to the suggested dosage on the label. If you notice no beneficial effects, say, within several weeks, add more – but do it gradually.

The best form to take vitamins is via the multiple vitamin tablet. This may be supplemented by additional, separate vitamin tablets for nutrients which either are not found, or are only present in insignificant amounts, in the multiple vitamin formula. *Always read the label on any vitamin tablet bottle carefully both for contents and other useful information.*

Please note that while vitamin pills may be catalysts that trigger rejuvenation and healing of illness, they may also create a dependency or 'vitamin addiction.' If this occurs, a 'withdrawal reaction' – along with the return of original symptoms – may temporarily arise when vitamin pill intake is stopped or even reduced.

If you notice any negative effects upon beginning taking vitamin pills, you are advised to test (by avoiding first one, then another, supplement until you get a distinct improvement or other indication) to see which of the supplements may be causing the problem. For this reason you may wish to use separate pills for each vitamin, rather than taking a particularly powerful multiple vitamin and mineral tablet. But please remember: *fresh foods grown locally are your best source of vitamins and other nutritional needs.*

Furthermore, it is easy to become too enthusiastic about taking nutritional supplements. Most people have been taught in school that the body simply 'throws off' excess nutrients. But modern doctors and scientists now find that this is not necessarily true – esp. for 'fat-soluble' vitamins (vitamins A, D, E, etc.). They tend to lodge themselves in the body's fat cells.

Common symptoms of excessive vitamin intake (vitaminosis) may include nausea, diarrhea, rashes, etc. Such problems occur most frequently with excesses of niacin, vitamin A and vitamin D.

Not only excess nutrients, but even reputedly beneficial foods – such as 'harmless' parsley – can be the source of unpleasant health problems when consumed to excess. The phrase, *more is better than less and sooner is better than later*, might apply to money and success, but not in the self-treatment of arthritis.

Fast 'cures' for dis-ease that has taken a long time to 'grow' and to manifest its symptoms and effects are highly suspect. Such healing processes appear to be contradictory to the laws of nature.

Preventive and/or Therapeutic Minerals and Other Supplements

Not only vitamins, but various essential minerals and elements are often depleted as arthritis develops and expands. Or their deficiency may cause arthritic symptoms to manifest themselves. In good health the body-mind actually manufactures these (as well as vitamins) from a wide variety of stimulants or sources, as mentioned above, through a miraculous process called 'biological transmutation' (described more completely in BIOLOGICAL TRANSMUTATIONS, by Dr. L. Kervran, Swan House Publishing Co., Brooklyn, N.Y.).

Among their many functions, minerals – even trace elements – are absolutely crucial in restoring and maintaining the delicate electrolytic balance of the body. When even small deficiencies of the following are present, serious consequences can occur in the electro-chemical system.

With the following minerals and trace elements – as with vitamins – fresh fruits and vegetables are your best source of most minerals (dolomite being the exception – this must be obtained from a health-food store). Please remember: nutritional supplements should only be used temporarily (maximum of six months to a year) to bridge the gap between the present diet and a better way of eating.

The following supplements (the most important of which are underlined) appear to help relieve the mineral deficiencies suffered by arthritic people:

* * <u>dolomite</u> (provides necessary magnesium and calcium – an arthritic person needs up to 500 Mg. daily of each mineral;
* * <u>calcium</u> (be sure to complement with equal amounts of magnesium);
* * hydrogen;
* * potassium;
* * sulphur;
* * bromelain (pineapple enzyme);
* * hydrochloric acid (HCL);
* * selenium;
* * sodium (through vegetables and herbs, not table salt);
* * iodine;
* * zinc (esp. psoriatic arthritis).

* (Reminder: before self-prescribing *any* nutritional supplement, it is wise to be professionally tested to make sure a deficiency – even a slight deficiency – exists.)

There are literally hundreds of 'folk' remedies for relieving arthritis and most of them 'work' – at least temporarily for some people. They wouldn't persist if they didn't bring somebody good results. The most popular of these remedies are simple to use and also help to restore many of the necessary minerals and elements to an arthritic system.

One such remedy is to mix – then drink – *epsom salts and cream of tartar in a glass of water* (a small amount of each, begin with half a teaspoon, or so, taken twice daily).

Another simple technique – wearing a *copper wire bracelet or anklet* – appears to have an electrolytic balancing effect on certain arthritis sufferers' systems. However, copper is a highly active and potentially toxic metal, and non-arthritic people should generally avoid wearing this metal. It is easily absorbed through the skin and may actually create pain in the joints of an otherwise healthy person.

A third popular remedy is to mix apple cider vinegar and raw honey – about a tablespoonful of each – into a glass of water, then drink it like a 'cocktail' several times daily. This should only be used cautiously (if at all) by vegetarians, but may be used more freely by slaughtered-food eaters.

But there is one additional supplement – iron – which should be *avoided* by arthritic individuals, especially those who suffer from *rheumatoid* arthritis. This is because iron tends to aggravate existing arthritis, making it more painful.

Preventive and/or Therapeutic Herbs and Other Natural 'Medicines'

Relieving and healing your arthritis may *begin* with changes in the diet, but there is more to self-healing with this ACUGENICS Program than simply adding 'good' foods to, and subtracting 'bad' ones from your diet. Another important aspect in treating your arthritis is the proper use of herbs and medicinal spices.

Like good food and nutritional supplements, herbal remedies appear to stimulate the appropriate organs, causing them to gradually self-correct and balance (heal) themselves.

There are literally hundreds of thousands of medicinal plants (some Oriental healers say *every* plant or flower has a medicinal value) and there are probably hundreds of such 'people-proven' healing flowers, leaves and roots that are specifically beneficial for arthritis sufferers.

But the following plant substances are relatively easy to obtain and yet have many enthusiastic proponents, both in the East and the West. Unless otherwise specified, these herbs and spices should be taken as a *tea* or *infusion*. They should be consumed several times a day, after being steeped for a minimum of 30 minutes in a covered glass, clay or ceramic – *not metal* – pot. Don't throw any herbal tea away: instead drink it cool, at room temperature. Use it instead of water or other, less-healthful beverages, such as coffee or soft drinks, whenever possible.

If you find there are several of these herbal teas you like, mix them. The most experienced herbalists usually suggest using blends of three, four or even five (but not more than five) herbs together for chronic problems.

Used alone and without other therapeutic practices, herbal therapy usually takes several months for satisfying results to occur. But when used in conjunction with other remedies and avoidances in this ACUGENICS Program, they become important natural supplements to accelerate your self-health program.

As with 'medicinal' fruits and vegetables, the best herbs for any ailment – including arthritis – are thought to grow near the sufferer's own home. First select from the following herbs those that are native to your area (within 50 miles), rather than seeking out the more foreign or exotic herbal remedies. Your county agriculture agent (or other official in charge of your local area's agricultural needs) is a useful source of that information.

If local herbs don't bring relief, then try some (or all) of the others. All of the following should be easily available either at a local health-food store or by mail. Check any popular health magazine for mail-order sources of herbal remedies. (Note: more in-depth discussion of the most popular herbal remedies, their uses and other important information will be found in THE G-JO

INSTITUTE MANUAL OF MEDICINAL HERBS, available from this publisher.

Here are some of the most popular herbs for self-treating arthritis:

* ginseng (males only – tends to make females too angry);
* black cohosh;
* sarsaparilla;
* birch leaves;
* yucca;
* valerian (use cautiously);
* buckthorn bark;
* dandelion;
* goldenseal;
* peppermint;
* ragwort;
* mountain flax;
* chaparral;
* nettles;
* skullcap;
* juniper berries;
* ginger (esp. fresh root);
* mistletoe;
* poke berries;
* sassafras;
* fenugreek;
* celery (used as a strong tea or infusion);
* peach tree leaves (esp. for gout);
* slippery elm;
* burdock;
* yarrow;
* comfrey (esp. root; leaves may be used as a poultice – see Section III);
* rosemary;
* sage.

There are a number of other edibles – that is, spices or cooking aids and such – which are very helpful in relieving and reversing arthritis . . . when used in conjunction with the other methods described herein. These should be used in moderation, of course – somewhere between the small doses of herbs, usually, and the larger servings of staples. They include:

* garlic (do not overuse);
* onions (do not overuse);
* basil;
* fennel;
* horseradish;
* oregano;
* lecithin (available from health food stores);
* capsicum (cayenne);
* sea water (2-3 Tbsp. daily);
* brewer's yeast (careful of allergy);
* chives;
* peanut and/or olive oil (cold-pressed – available at health food stores – both for cooking and with salads);
* raw cream (if you can find it).

However, at least several of these substances rank high on the list of potentially-abusive or -allergic foods (notably garlic, onions, cayenne and brewer's yeast). Please pay particular attention to notice if any adverse effects occur following their use.

One useful daily nutritional arthritis self-treatment program, which is to be used in conjunction with other methods and techniques described below, calls for the following:

1. One Tbsp. of cold-pressed peanut oil (mixed with non-citrus fruit or vegetable juice);

2. 1000 Mg. <u>calcium</u> plus 500 Mg. <u>magnesium</u> (or equivalent amount of <u>dolomite</u>);

3. <u>Alfalfa</u> – in tablet form (up to 24 tablets daily) or, better, a good handful of alfalfa sprouts;

4. Up to one half lb. of <u>cherries</u> daily (fresh or unsweetened canned or frozen); may gradually be decreased to twice weekly; and if cherries are not available, <u>strawberries</u> may be substituted;

5. <u>Vitamin A</u> – up to 25,000 I.U. (optional);

6. <u>Niacin/vitamin B_3</u> (either as nicotinic acid – which causes a 'flush' – or as niacinamide, up to a maximum of two grams daily, divided into four equal doses to be taken at mealtime); also take an equal amount of vitamin C, but reduce or eliminate step #6 if queasiness or nausea occur (step #6 is particularly helpful for arthritis of the knee);

7. Vitamin B_6/pyridoxine – males take 200-600 Mg.; females take 300-800 Mg. (esp. for arthritis of hands and fingers);

8. Vitamin B_{12}/cobalamin – 1000 mcg. (esp. for bursitis – vegetarians, be sure this is not from animal sources);

9. Vitamin B_5/pantothenic acid – try 100 Mg. daily maximum;

10. Vitamin C – 250 Mg.;

11. Vitamin E – 45 I.U.;

12. Selenium – 100 mcg.

As with all programs that depend on nutritional supplements, the above program should be considered a temporary 'bridge' between the present diet and a more healthful, future move toward the recommendations described earlier.

29

Section III:
Non-Nutritional Therapies

There are several non-nutritional deficiencies commonly found in arthritis sufferers. Their remedies will be discussed in this section. Several of these common deficiencies include:

* low blood oxygen levels;
* lack of regular exercise;
* having no method for expressing 'hidden' (or restrained) anger and resentment, a method that is both direct yet nondestructive.

As hidden or unresolved emotions and other abuses build, their 'results' – in the form of toxins or 'poisons' – tend to lodge themselves in the joints and other susceptible parts of the body of those who are so predisposed: that is a capsule view of arthritis.

Stimulate and restore balance to the malfunctioning organs and joints, and release the abuses that feed arthritis – then the body-mind begins healing itself and arthritis reverses itself. This is a capsule view of the ACUGENICS method of relieving and healing arthritis.

There are a number of self-health methods for stimulating, 'cleansing' and 'balancing' the malfunctioning organs, aside from the previously mentioned nutritional means. The most important of these self-applied therapies are:

* <u>moderate exercise</u>;

* breath control;
* self-psychotherapy;
* temperature changes (esp. heat);
* prayer, meditation and visualization;
* acupressure (acupuncture without needles) and
  other self-massage techniques.

Some Thoughts on Exercise . . .

Because of its beneficial effects on the liver, some form
of *regular*, gentle-to-moderate (and perhaps occasionally
vigorous) exercise program is vital to an arthritis
sufferer. Exercise helps cleanse the entire system – via
perspiration and other excretory functions – as well as
easing the pain (because of the temporary electro-
chemical changes that occur following even brief
exercise).

The ideal exercise program for arthritis sufferers is
based on *gentle stretching and movement*. For many
arthritis sufferers this is all they can manage, anyway.
But under any circumstances, it is always wise to avoid
harsh, violent exercise or sports.

Focus, instead, should be on a kind of *slow*, free-form
or unstructured *dancing* – done preferably outside in the
sunlight (wearing only light cotton clothing, if possible) – until a light sheen of perspiration forms across
the brow and shoulders.

Ideally, this 'slow dance' should be done to the beat of
Gregorian chants or other church-like music. In fact, the
slower the movements, the better. As you move, grace is
less important than slow stretching – especially stretching the extremities (the fingers and even the toes, if you
can manage it). Each muscle should get some benefits
from the movement.

Doing this for just a few minutes a day is often

enough exercise to be energizing and invigorating. For many arthritis sufferers, freedom from pain is measured in minutes, not hours, and slow dance will often bring increasingly long spans of 'relief time' – especially when combined with other parts of this ACUGENICS Self-Health Program.

For many arthritis sufferers, *hatha yoga* and its numerous postures and poses (called *asanas*) brings at least temporary relief. If you follow the path of yoga, however, please be sure to allow yourself enough *rest time* between poses for the full benefits of this activity to occur. With hatha yoga (one of the 16 types of yoga in East Indian philosophy), it is again the slow stretching and contraction of the muscles – as well as the flexing of the joints – which allows certain 'toxic' biochemicals to be *released*. But it is the *resting* that allows them to be *purged* into the excretory system or 'neutralized' and resorbed elsewhere.

Hatha yoga is a way of life. There are numerous books on the subject and nearly every town and city now has yoga classes – often in conjunction with local colleges, churches or adult education centers. These classes are the best places to learn the special 'broad-spectrum' healing postures and poses. But it is vital to remember that yoga is neither a sport nor a test of strength and endurance. You only need to hold the pose long enough to feel a slight sense of exertion – this indicates these trapped biochemicals have been released.

Holding a yogic posture longer than necessary, or 'competing' – either against yourself or someone in a yoga class to see who can hold a difficult pose the longest – is totally contrary to the nature and purpose of this otherwise useful technique.

But the most useful exercise clearly is brisk *walking* (usually 300-400 steps a day is enough, especially if you are a vegetarian). Briskly walking even these few steps a day stimulates virtually every organ muscle and joint in the body. It produces a prompt feeling of well-being that continues, in many cases, for several hours or more.

Bicycling and *swimming* are other very beneficial moderate exercises, too. However, in all forms of exercise, please remember that it is the *quality* – not the quantity – of the exercise that counts. It is more important that *all* parts of the system (especially the joints of the extremities) receive *some* flexion, than for a few parts to receive strenuous activity while others remain dormant.

Try to combine gently shaking and flexing your wrists, fingers and ankles with whatever exercise you do. Even cracking your knuckles – if you suffer from regular pain in them – might be a good form of stretching and flexion (it also helps release stress that is 'stored' there). And with a little forethought, nearly any activity you do can be made into some beneficial kind of exercise or therapy. Even watching TV can be therapeutic . . . if you combine it with rocking in a rocking chair (a very good exercise, incidentally, especially for those with arthritis in the hips, back or knees). All it takes is desire and a bit of imagination. (Note: a more complete fitness program – suitable for people of all ages and in nearly any state of health – is found in this author's *How to Get Fit – and Stay Fit – The Acugenic Method*, available from the same publisher.)

Simply keeping active socially often provides enough exercise; especially if you combine walking, dancing or some other techniques with your social life. Staying socially active has numerous other benefits too, emotional as well as physical (not the least of which is helping the sufferer to avoid thinking about himself or his suffering).

Even if you don't have many friends – a common

complaint among arthritis sufferers – start new projects . . . take some time at least once a week to do some kind of volunteer or service work . . . try *new* activities! Arthritis is as much a point of view as it is a dysfunction of the organs and glands.

As mentioned earlier, the lungs – in conjunction with the liver and kidneys – are said to play an important role in the process of arthritis. In fact, according to many healers throughout history, the lungs play a rich part in the creation, maintenance and destruction of *most* diseases.

Of all the major organs, the lungs are the most easily 'reached' for self-therapy. And the therapy itself is very simple: *deep, controlled breathing done in series, several times a day*! At the most, it takes only several minutes and may be done anywhere and nearly any time.

Any kind of deep breathing exercise will be helpful, as long as you follow the rules below. First, take at least ten deep breaths – filling your lungs to capacity – then exhaling as deeply as you can. Next, always breathe 'into' and 'from' your lower abdomen (that is, imagine your inhaled breath traveling to – then being exhaled from – the area about two inches below the navel).

And finally, unless specified to the contrary, always breathe through the *nostrils*, not the mouth. To make this nasal breathing process technique even more effective, roll the tip of your tongue upward into the roof of your mouth as often as possible. Eventually, this may automatically become your normal way of breathing while at rest – a particularly healthful way, according to Oriental doctor-philosophers.

There are specific ways of breathing deeply which are more effective (in improving the blood's oxygen level) than others. One excellent method of deep breathing – one that has been practiced by disciples of hatha yoga for many centuries – consists simply of a '1-2-1-2' cycle.

This means that for every one count of inhaled or exhaled breath you take, you hold it for two (at both the 'top' and 'bottom' of the cycle). For example: begin your breathing cycle by totally emptying your lungs; then gradually (with your tongue tucked into the roof of your mouth) draw in a long breath – drawing it into as 'low in your abdomen' as you can, through your nostrils – for, say, a count of five. Then hold your breath for a count of ten (that is, two times the five-count on your inhale). Then exhale on a measured, gradual basis for another five count . . . and sit quietly with your lungs emptied for another ten count. Repeat this ten times each session for at least two sessions daily, if possible.

If this causes too much strain, reduce the in-out count to a point that is comfortable. Conversely, if you don't feel a bit uncomfortable with this cycle, do a 6-12-6-12 – or even longer – count, to the point of feeling slight exertion. The goal is to increase your 'lung power.'

Within several weeks of consciously controlling your breath in this manner, you'll actually find yourself breathing more deeply and regularly, feeling more calm and less prone to anger, and being better able to keep 'centered' in previously emotion-filled situations.

One interesting variation of this process suggests reading as much of a newspaper article as you can on your out-breath (and, of course, trying to empty your lungs as completely as possible in the process). Your in-breath should be as deep and slow as you can manage.

Another variation is the *cleansing* – actually hyperventilating – breath cycle. This is simply rapid, deep breathing (most people can't reach a count of ten without feeling very lightheaded at first), done several times a day. This variation is good to do just *occasionally* and only while you are seated.

Still another effective breath control method involves

closing one side of the nostril with a thumb or finger on the in-breath, then opening that side and closing the other nostril with a fingertip on the out-breath. It requires more concentration and control to avoid rushing or panicking in the process.

But the normal deep, slow-breathing technique described at first is quite adequate for greatly increasing your lung-power and adding benefits to your other self-health efforts and techniques.

With any of the aforementioned deep-breathing techniques, the ultimate purpose is both relief as well as retraining yourself to breathe properly. Very few people actually take more than very shallow breaths, except under rare circumstances – yawning, smoking a cigarette or after intense physical activity, for instance.

Remember: practicing your deep breathing exercises in the beginning of your self-health program is essential. Later, after you make several weeks of conscious effort, it will begin to become a normal activity and eventually become a regular part of your breathing cycle.

There are several other important external therapies which are at least temporarily beneficial to many arthritis sufferers.

Oil balms and massages have long been a favorite of self-healers for speedy, effective relief. One popular Oriental over-the-counter remedy is called *Tiger Balm* – a pleasantly scented wax-like substance – which millions of Easterners use for many ailments . . . including arthritis-type pains. It is available in most Oriental grocery shops and many health-food stores. Its benefits are not imaginary – this remarkable salve wouldn't be so popular if they were.

Another 'balm' is DMSO, a veterinary substance used as a liniment for horses and other large animals. Many individuals have found relief by using this potentially dangerous chemical substance. It is often available by mail or from health-food stores (in America) . . . but it should be used cautiously, and immediately be stopped or reduced if you notice adverse reactions. Begin by placing only a *tiny* amount on one small area of skin, to test for any unpleasant reactions.

Another potentially dangerous substance – *aconite liniment* – has a long history of bringing relief from arthritis. This liniment is prepared by 'marinating' four oz. of ground aconite (*Aconitum Napellus* or monkshood) root in one quart of strong (120 proof) vodka, in a warm place for several days (until it turns the color of dark tea).

Then rub a *small* amount of this (one tsp. maximum) into a test area until dry. Cover that area with flannel and let it stand overnight, then wash the test area in the morning. Discontinue its use if a rash or similar reaction occurs. Avoid being chilled when using this liniment, and *do not use it if there is a known heart condition*.

If no adverse reaction occurs, gradually increase area of usage – but since this is a powerful and potentially dangerous substance, please use only under medical supervision (at least, in the beginning).

Of the various oils often recommended, three – *olive, peanut and castor oil* – appear most frequently in natural healing 'prescriptions.' Their use is simple enough: just massage the selected oil into the sore areas, especially the most painful joints. However, when using castor oil, it is best to *avoid inflamed joints or other areas*.

While these oils may be used cold (at room temperature), when the oily area is covered with a layer of cloth and a heating pad to make a *radiant oil treatment*, their effectiveness is greatly increased.

The greater the arthritic suffering, the longer these radiant oil packs should stay in place – perhaps up to several hours, in some cases. They are best done during a time of relaxation – say, just before an afternoon nap or at bedtime.

Another effective remedy using heat is to simply take a long, hot bath (a steam bath or turkish bath is even better) – then quickly follow that with a *brief* cold shower. And since warmth seems so important in the treatment of arthritis, try *sleeping in a sleeping bag* to maintain a uniform sense of warmth throughout the night. In fact, artificially increasing the body temperature (by any means) to at least 103°F. on a regular (say twice weekly) basis is said to have very beneficial effects.

Further still, apply *hot paraffin wax* to affected areas. Heat the waxy substance in an old saucepan to a fluid consistency, then dab the paraffin wax onto affected area(s). Peel off (for reheating) after the wax has cooled and hardened. Store in the saucepan and repeat the treatment twice daily (or more).

Sunlight has a beneficial effect, too. If possible, expose your face (or as much of the body as possible) to direct sunlight for at least 15 minutes daily – perhaps while doing your slow dancing routine out-of-doors.

Keep your eyes open when looking toward the sun. Do not look directly into the sun, of course, but look as near to it as possible until discomfort occurs, then look slightly away. This is a very effective way to accelerate healing since it has a profound effect on the liver (the eyes are also thought to be 'connected' to the liver, according to Oriental health philosophy).

At the other end of the temperature spectrum, *ice* – massaged symptomatically on affected areas (esp. the knees) – often provides equally pleasant, if temporary, relief . . . after the initial discomfort is overcome. Use this ice massage symptomatically. Hint: freeze a rubber glove full of water to make an 'ice hand,' then use that to rub onto affected areas (after stripping the glove off the frozen 'hand').

Sexual orgasm or ejaculation is one of the most powerful ways to bring temporary relief of arthritic pain and suffering (because of the powerful 'draining' effect on the liver). If necessary, masturbation can bring nearly as much relief as normal coitus.

The external use of herbs – especially as *poultices* (packs of crushed leaves or other vegetable substances that are bound onto an affected area for up to several hours) – is an art that is returning to popularity after being mostly ignored by Westerners for many decades.

The most common way to make a poultice is to first crush an herbal root, leaves or complete plant – *comfrey* (especially the leaves) is one of the best for arthritic suffering (see section on herbal remedies for others). Then either place this mash directly on the skin or (more commonly) on a light cotton cloth (perhaps a piece of bedsheet, and fold it over into an 'envelope' or package). Then bind or wrap the pack onto the affected area with another piece of cloth. Let it stay in place for as long as possible.

Many different plants and herbs have been successfully used for poultices – even *common grass*! – so don't be afraid to experiment. Remember: many natural healers claim that the nearer to one's home the therapeutic plant or herb grows, the more beneficial it is. Always first try the earlier-listed herbs; or ask your local agricultural agent or government-provided home economist for that information.

As with an oil or balm, a heating pad placed around or atop any poultice may increase its beneficial effects. Let it stay in place for up to several hours, if possible, and repeat up to several times daily.

Learning to directly – but nondestructively – confront important sources of emotional irritants that trigger your suffering may be even more important than exercise or diet control. Not surprisingly, it may also be more difficult to do. But until you do find a way to deal with these hidden or stashed emotions, any other therapy will generally only have limited results.

If you are an arthritic woman, this may mean confronting a husband, son and/or father. If you are an arthritic man, it may mean confronting an employer (or a wife). In either case, it raises a very uncomfortable possibility – that person may either be very hurt or even say back to you: 'If you don't like it here, get out!'

Furthermore, even if the situation applies to you and you can muster up the courage to confront this situation, there are still two other possible problems. First, *you* – not the other person(s) – may be the real problem. Many or most of the harsh emotions we ever feel are really *not* justified, but simply are misunderstandings, old points of view and gross misconceptions. And like a blazing fire, these feelings are fed and fueled by the food we eat and the lifestyle we live.

Fortunately, as you improve your diet along the above selected guidelines – especially as you eliminate salt, slaughtered foods, sugar and alcohol – the strength, length (of time), fiery quality and depth of destructive emotions is dramatically reduced. And it happens rather quickly – usually within several weeks of these dietary eliminations.

But the second problem may be this: even if your feelings *may* be justified reactions to important people in your life, and even if you *do* take all the steps suggested in this ACUGENICS Program, you may well be dealing with insensitive people who wouldn't understand (or perhaps wouldn't even care) what you're talking about.

It is in cases such as this that psychotherapy or self-development seminars may be most helpful. But this can be an expensive, long drawn out process – and it usually requires participation of all family members to be its most effective. On the other hand, there are several 'self-psychotherapy' techniques you can apply to release some of this repressed emotional pressure and distress.

'Psychotherapy' is basically the verbalization of conscious fears and other strong feelings – with the hope of finding subconscious keys . . . emotional relief . . . and solutions to the underlying problems.

We can, and often do, accomplish this in many ways: we complain about our problems to family or friends . . . we get angry and have arguments . . . we may seek professional or religious counseling . . . we may even turn to astrology, psychics or other sources of real or questionable merit.

But each of these ways has its drawbacks. Some methods only vent emotions without helping us find solutions. Others are bizarre, often worthless and occasionally harmful. And nearly always, they bring someone else into the picture.

Yet our problems are our own: we created them (by our interpretation or misinterpretation of events and situations – often in childhood – as well as by our actions); and only we, alone, can solve them. Self-psychotherapy helps perform that function by *revealing our problem(s) to ourselves*, then *pointing the way(s) to their solutions*.

Self-psychotherapy is essentially *talking to yourself* (either in thought or by actual words) . . . but in a detached and self-observant manner. It means becoming your own counselor – no easy task, but made much easier with one or more of the following techniques.

As mentioned earlier, one of the best techniques is *keeping a daily journal or diary*. If you find that too hard or inconvenient, take a few minutes each day to *talk to a wall*. Or, better, to a mirror. Not just *think* to a wall or mirror, but openly *verbalize* your thoughts and feelings as best as possible, to your 'wailing wall.'

Actually getting 'stashed words' out into the open has a profoundly cathartic and uplifting effect . . . sometimes shockingly so! As words begin to tumble forth, it is not uncommon for a train of thought to release feelings of which you were not even consciously aware.

If you have a guru or spiritual master (such as Jesus), it may help greatly to have His picture placed in front of you to look at and speak to. If not, perhaps a pretty painting or photograph – even a picture of yourself to look at while you speak.

To spur the process along, try finishing each thought with the question 'so what?' or 'so what's the worst thing that can happen?'; then try to answer that question, verbalizing your answer to your wall or mirror. Check the answer against reality – many of our worries seem actually silly when revealed to the light of reality by this verbalization process.

Openly verbalizing and/or writing down your feelings and complaints releases the pressures that drive harsh emotions deeper within you. These buried emotions would otherwise overstimulate your 'arthritis control organs,' especially the lungs and liver, thus tending to manifest this distress later as pain and suffering.

Keeping a daily journal also helps to stimulate important sights and self-revelations. Your diary also provides you with a permanent, ongoing record of your exciting voyage toward self-health and well-being.

It cannot be repeated often enough: in virtually every case of arthritis, it is the sufferer's own *attitude* that is at the root of the problem. Reviewing your daily record will help reveal to you where the problems lie – and often point the way to their solutions.

Remember: your journal may well become a revealer of 'trigger foods' that actually cause the most serious bouts of suffering. Taking a few minutes to list each food and beverage consumed during a meal will almost invariably highlight surprising connections between certain foods and suffering. Hint: look back two or three days after a particularly severe bout of pain to locate key trigger foods.

Meditation Plus Specific Prayers and/or Visualizations

Prayerful meditation is an especially powerful technique (which might be considered another self-psychotherapy method) whose benefits and results could fill several books by themselves. The ACUGENICS method involves three specific steps to achieve the most effective results:

1. Prayer
2. Meditation
3. Visualization

This prayerful meditation is best done *when you have the least time to do it* (e.g., when you're rushed or under stress – the times that anger, resentment and/or hostility are most likely to be at their most intense). A second good time to use this process is at bedtime, in the moments just between awakeness and dropping off to sleep. These few minutes are when the subconscious mind (and the spiritual part of oneself) are most easily reached and 'controlled' – see below. Another good time for performing this prayerful meditation (which only takes a few minutes, with practice) is just before arising. If possible, awaken 15 minutes earlier than usual. But if you have to rush through the process, don't do this exercise. It's better to arise relaxed than to feel tense and hurried just to meditate. In fact it can't be done.

You are trying to reach – or to utilize – that special 'bridge' state which occurs in the near-selfless time between being awake and being asleep. It is the time we are most free of our egos and, because pain and distress are eased by selflessness, also the time we are most free from our suffering. Following each of these steps in their order, you will be able to put yourself into this remarkably pleasant and relaxed state.

Begin by directing your prayer to God or Universal Spirit (or whatever 'higher' Force you believe exists within/outside of yourself). Urge It to reveal to you in your meditation (or in whatever fashion It chooses), the source of – *and the way to release* – any hostile, aggressive feelings you may (or may not) sense you have at the root of your illness.

In your prayer, it is important to ask for help in revealing to yourself your *own* part in the process. Ask to be presented with ways for best dealing with your anger in the highest, most loving method for all parties concerned. Pray for help in recognizing and fully appreciating that it is anger, hostility and resentment – created and perpetuated only by you, allowed into your body-mind *only* with your permission – that is the key to your suffering.

Upon completing your prayer, become meditative. That is, relax and try letting go of any 'rational' thoughts – but don't slip into sleep. A good technique is to quietly whisper the number 'one' or the word 'ommm' over and over. This will help focus your attention and keep you 'here.'

Don't be concerned if you can't seem to stay focused and attentive: that will come with practice. A simple trick to instantly 'deepen' your meditative state is to cross your closed eyes (as if you were looking at the tip of your nose or the point between but above the eyebrows) while silently repeating your single word – it should help you stay centered.

To further deepen and intensify this pleasant, relaxed

state, mentally count from ten to one (or vice-versa), releasing any accumulated stress and tension from a specific area of the body with each number counted. For example, when thinking of the number 'ten,' focus on relaxing the feet and toes; with number 'nine,' the lower legs and knees; with 'eight,' the thighs, etc. To make the relaxation even more complete, first tightly clench all your muscles for a few moments. Then release and do your 'countdown.'

Finally, when it feels right, make positive use of this relaxed state by beginning to visualize the negative or painful qualities of your arthritis as a clear, mental picture. Perhaps imagine your stiff and sore joints as being bound in hardening cement; then visualize this substance falling off in tiny particles, and imagine your system breaking up and purging these deposits that now bind your joints and make them painful to move.

Or visualize your most tender and painful joints as being 'glued' tightly together. But as soon as you can 'see' that in your mind, visualize a gentle, warm solvent starting to flow in your system to dissolve that 'glue.'

To replace this glue or cement, feel love, light, warmth and relaxation entering either through your head or the bottom of your feet, moving steadily toward – and into – your heart. Let some of this feeling seep outwards, to the tips of your fingers and toes ... and all areas between.

Then send that same love, light and warmth outward, from your heart, beyond your painful joints or bones, toward those people closest to you – especially those whom you feel may be most directly 'responsible' for your arthritis – even if they are deceased! As you 'broadcast' this loving warmth, feel fresh, vital tissue replacing the old, cemented tissue and bony areas.

This technique may be done sitting or lying down – whichever is most comfortable or convenient. However, as mentioned above, you should not be so comfortable as to fall asleep or even become too drowsy. This defeats the purpose. If you tend to fall asleep easily, definitely do this technique while sitting in a straight-backed chair.

As with breathing techniques, there are many possible variations of that third and final step – visualization. Another good way involves first relaxing the area above, between and below the eyes (liver- and kidney-related areas, according to Oriental doctors), and along the sides of the mouth (lung-related).

Then focus 'relaxation' (or 'send healing energy') to the liver area (just below the right breast, above the bottom of the rib cage), while repeating to your subconscious part an instruction to calm and restore proper functioning of the liver.

Then focus on your entire chest, especially the lungs, trying to become aware of any hostility and angry words that might be stored there. Now visualize those words shrinking smaller and smaller into tiny motes of dust floating into the middle of your lungs. Then, when they are small enough, see/feel them being exhaled into the universe for purification (you may actually have coughing spasms in the beginning of this practice).

Finally, move your focus to the lower middle back – the kidney area – and try to feel your kidneys 'unkink' and ease any tension stored there as you send radiant warmth and light to them.

The variations are endless. And if you already have a meditative or self-relaxation technique, these are good ways to expand. But whatever method you use, always make sure that you close your meditation (or awaken yourself) with the suggestion that you forgive yourself, forgive those who are linked to your arthritis, and feel love for all – *especially for yourself!*

Important 'Acupressure' Methods and Techniques

Acupressure (acupuncture without needles) is an ancient Oriental self-health art that relies on thumb- or finger-tip pressure to stimulate (by deep, specific massage) the body's tiny therapeutic points. This is by far the most powerful and effective self-health technique known to man, and is a key ingredient of this ACUGENICS Arthritis Self-Health Program.

There are more than 1200 of these pinhead-sized acupuncture points on the body, of which more than 200 are highly pressure-responsive. This drugless technique is extremely effective for both relieving pain quickly (usually within 10 or 15 *seconds*) and for helping to stimulate the body-mind's own self-healing mechanisms.

This technique – which is called 'G-Jo' (simplified acupressure) – is a three-step process: first, you must *find the right point*; second, you must *'trigger' (stimulate) the point properly*; and third, you then *stimulate the identical point on the opposite side of the body* (if applicable – generally speaking, points on the ear are not stimulated bilaterally, but rather only the most tender point(s) on one ear are selected for acupressure stimulation . . . see details below).

To find the right pressure point, turn to the illustrations in the following pages of this book and begin deeply probing those areas of your body that correspond to the illustrations. You are looking for tender 'ouch points' – those that feel like a toothache or pinched nerve when pressed or probed.

You must probe as deeply as you can (except in the ear – different instructions, below), pressing with up to 20 lbs. of fingertip pressure (use a bathroom scale to see just how much 20 lbs. of pressure is). Use the tip (not the pad or fleshy part) of your thumb or the bent knuckle of

47

your index finger, if you have long thumbnails. If you are elderly or don't have quite enough strength, you must use the eraser tip of a pencil (but don't press too deeply or you might bruise yourself).

When both finding and triggering points on the ear, use either the non-lighting end of a wooden matchstick or a toothpick whose point has been clipped off with a nail-clipper. Acupressure points in the ear are somewhat more difficult to locate (often, you might need a partner to find these points the first few times). But they are extremely effective in bringing relief and even promoting self-healing.

Stimulate the most tender of these points deeply enough for the point to feel quite sensitive, using a digging, goading kind of fingertip (or matchstick) massage; do this for up to four minutes on either side of your body (other than the ear), until you feel an 'acupressure reaction.' This is a feeling of warmth, clamminess, perspiration or such – usually across the forehead, shoulders, neck or cheeks.

Often, just a few seconds of acupressure stimulation is enough to produce this reaction . . . and to produce relief. These points may be stimulated four or five times a day, until the tenderness at the point(s) disappears or is greatly reduced (this may take several weeks or longer).

The exact way G-Jo works is still a mystery – or at least a controversial issue between traditional Eastern healers and many of their Western counterparts. But its results are undeniable – G-Jo really works within minutes . . . especially for minor ailments or discomfort. To a Westerner accustomed to relying on drugs and medications for symptomatic relief, the speed at which this happens is nothing less than astounding!

These points will vary slightly from person to person, but a few moments of fingertip probing will quickly uncover your own sensitive ouch point – it will be unmistakable after you know what these points feel like when contacted. Just feel around for the 'ouch!'

When you find one that is particularly sensitive, circle it on the illustrated pages of points below. Then use those points as your own, special 'acupressure formula' for the next several weeks, or so. Remember: when the tenderness disappears, you stop doing G-Jo.

All the G-Jo points are tiny – only about the size of a pinhead – so it may be a bit difficult to find a point, at first. But after you find several of them on your own body, you'll quickly recognize the characteristic twinge – which some people describe as feeling 'like a toothache or pinched nerve' – that only happens when a 'good' point is properly probed.

While you should begin by triggering both sides of the body identically, nearly always one side will be more tender than the other (often, but not always, the points on the right side will be more tender for females, while those on the left are more tender on males). The more sensitive side is usually the more effective, so you can spend a bit longer triggering it. This bilateral stimulation of the points helps to 'balance the body's energy between yin and yang (negative and positive bioelectrical potentials),' according to Oriental doctors, which is vital for long-term healing to occur.

Within humane limits, it is difficult to stimulate your own points too deeply (except for the ear, which should only be lightly stimulated); on the other hand, it is quite easy not to stimulate them deeply enough. And since each point is small – less than a centimeter or two in diameter – it is vital to be precise. Both the illustration and the printed instructions only give approximate locations. The 'loud' twinge of sensitivity is your true indicator.

Remember: in addition to the 'ouch,' a good point will often make you break out in an immediate flush of perspiration – or create a sudden sense of relaxation or feeling of warmth – when it's deeply stimulated. Then, too, you might experience a tingling sensation, or a sense of 'energy flowing'; you might even feel a bit faint, and have to sit down for a few minutes. In any event, it is always better to be relaxed when you use G-Jo – do it either seated or lying down.

While many points may beneficially affect a specific symptom, usually one or two points in particular will 'do the job' best. Stimulate the best (that is, usually the most tender) point(s) as soon as you notice the arthritic discomfort occur or return – this is very important, for the sooner G-Jo is begun, the better and more effective it is. You should get increasing spans of 'relief time' – time between necessary restimulations. This is a good indicator that you've found the right G-Jo point(s) for your symptom.

If you don't get prompt, satisfactory relief, it usually means one of several things:

1. You didn't find the right control point for that symptom – try another point;
2. You didn't stimulate a point, only *near* a point – did you feel the twinge of sensitivity when you probed and stimulated?
3. You didn't stimulate the point properly – did you use enough fingertip pressure? Did you stimulate long enough?
4. Your problem may be beyond the scope of G-Jo – seek professional attention (perhaps have acu*puncture* with needles performed).

However, acupressure should be avoided:

* If you are a chronic heart patient, especially if you wear a pacemaker or other artificial energy-regulating device;

* If you are a pregnant woman (especially beyond your third month of pregnancy);
* If you take regular or daily medication (other than an occasional aspirin) – acupressure and medications do not mix well, which is generally true of most forms of natural therapy . . . either use medicines or natural therapy, but do not use both unless suggested/approved by your doctor.

There are several other times when the use of these points should be temporarily avoided: within four hours of taking drugs, medications, alcohol or other intoxicants; within half an hour after taking a hot bath, eating a heavy meal or doing physical exercise; and avoid any of the suggested points that lie beneath a scar, mole, wart or other blemish.

In the beginning of acupressure self-treatment, it is not unusual to eventually produce a 'healing crisis' – a kind of deep cleansing that may manifest itself as a temporary change in the bowels, a mild fever, a feeling of lethargy, etc. Do not be discouraged by these phenomena (if they occur); keep triggering the most tender points until their tenderness fades. However, if these reactions become too intense, reduce – or temporarily discontinue – your acupressure until you feel better.

Normally, there is an underlying feeling of growing wellness, as if the healing crisis is a natural 'sloughing off' of bodily impurities. It is, in fact, a very encouraging feeling for most people . . . they can somehow sense the 'rightness' of it.

Acupressure should be used as supportive therapy with other self-health techniques – especially the avoidance of the above-described abusive foods or any known allergens. There are a number of acupressure points which may benefit a number of forms of arthritis. The following pressure points are mainly pain control points for general use – additionally, there are also points included that primarily affect specific areas, such as the hands, shoulders, etc. These may be used alone or in combination with the most tender 'general use' points – the key is to use the points that bring the most complete and long-lasting relief.

There are numerous other acupressure points for specific bodily areas covered in the THE NATURAL HEALER'S ACUPRESSURE HANDBOOK, VOLUME I: BASIC G-JO (or, for a complete healing program using acupressure, THE NATURAL HEALER'S ACUPRES- SURE HANDBOOK, VOLUME II: ADVANCED G-JO; both of which are available from the same publisher). Furthermore, there are complete acupressure healing systems in either hand and foot. These are completely described, and the acupressure points illustrated, in two of this author's other books: HOW TO HEAL YOUR- SELF USING HAND ACUPRESSURE; and HOW TO HEAL YOURSELF USING FOOT ACUPRESSURE (also available from the same publisher).

General Arthritis Acupressure Points

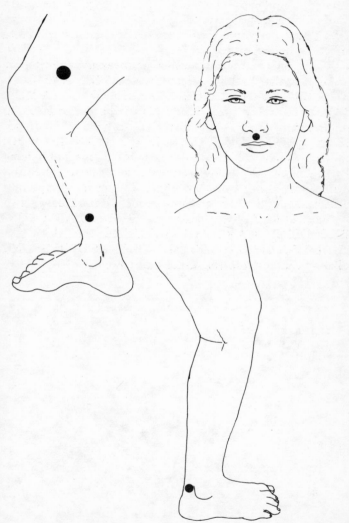

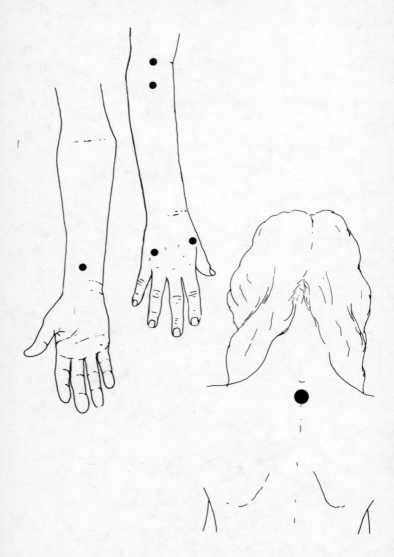

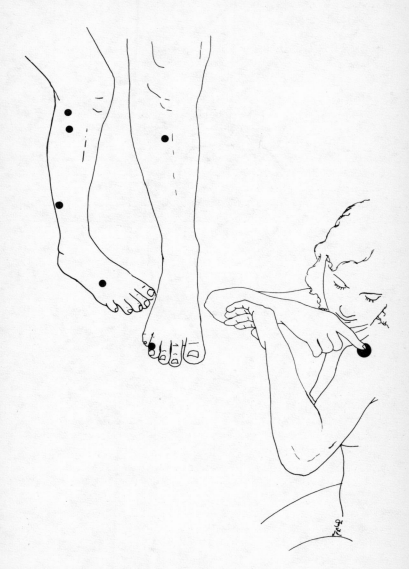

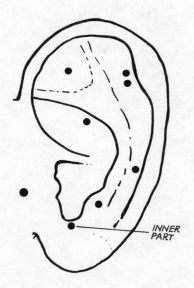

INNER
PART

Acupressure Points for Pain in the Elbows

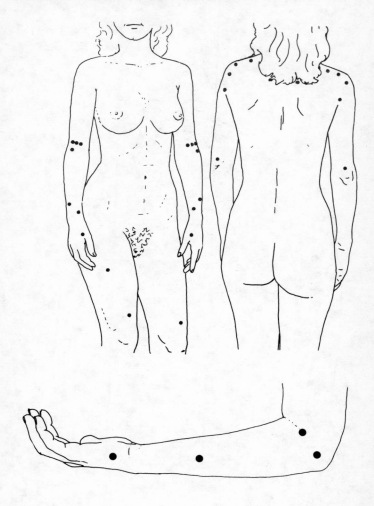

Acupressure Points for Pain in the Hands, Fingers and Wrist

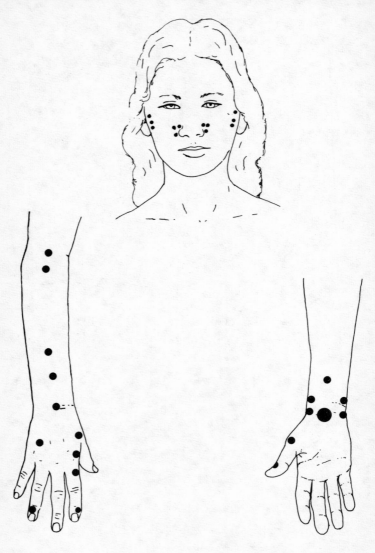

Acupressure Points for Pain in the Shoulders and Neck

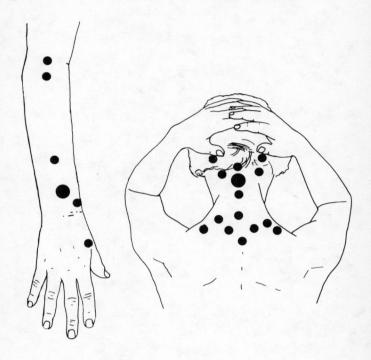

Acupressure Points for Pain in the Hips

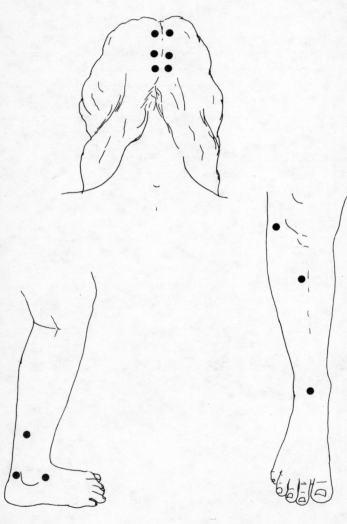

Acupressure Points for Pain in the Low Back

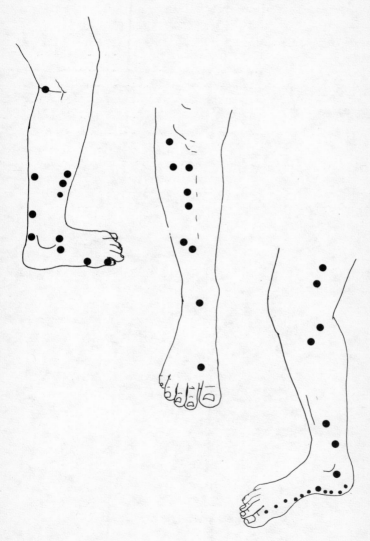

Acupressure Points for Pain in the Knees

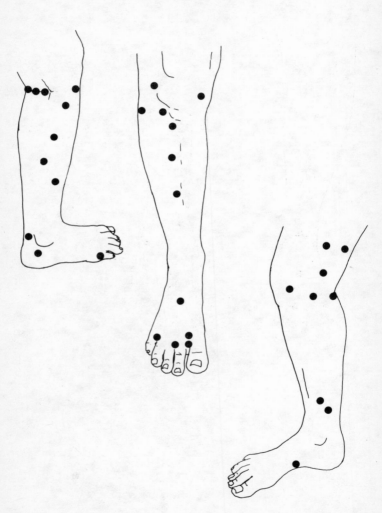

Acupressure Points for Pain in the Feet and Toes

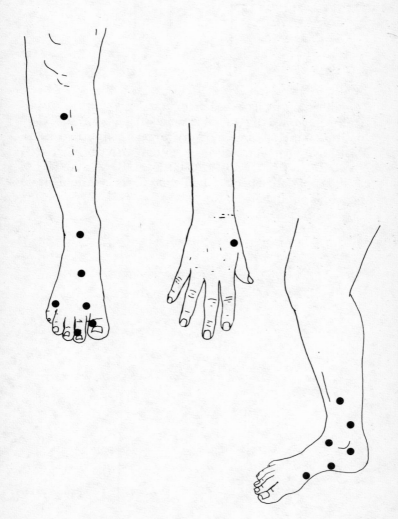

Section IV:
Recipes Using 'Arthritis-Fighting' Foods

The following recipes – each 'taste-tested' and enthusiastically endorsed by members and friends of the G-Jo Institute – include one or more 'arthritis-fighting' foods. Most have been selected from Gail Watson's COOKING NATURALLY FOR PLEASURE AND HEALTH (a cookbook of delicious, yet medicinal foods, available from the same publisher).

ARTHRITIS PROGRAM (MENU)

	Day 1	Day 2	Day 3	Day 4	Day 5	Day 6	Day 7
	Upon rising or ½ hour before breakfast: 1 small glass of fresh grapefruit juice, pineapple juice or diluted cherry juice; or fresh, raw vegetable juice (carrot, celery, tomato, etc.; or in combination with each other).						
BREAKFAST	Granola with Dried Fruit Almond Cream	Brown Rice Waffles with Homemade Applesauce	Cinnamon Oatmeal with Bananas and Yogurt	Brown Rice Cream Cereal and Fig Lassi	Strawberry Oatmeal Waffles with Strawberry Sauce	Millet-Sesame Cereal with Bananas Cashew Cream	Whole-Grain Pancakes with Cherry Sauce
MAIN MEAL	Corn Chowder Sauteed Parsnips & Carrots Lentil Vegie Loaf Rice Pudding	Carrot-Raisin Salad Endive Potatoes Tofu Croquettes Gravy #2 Pecan Pie	Watercress-String Bean Salad Tofu-Mushroom Stroganoff Strawberry Pie	Stuffed Beets Broccoli-Cauliflower Casserole Miso Gravy Sweet Yam Tarts	Tangy Apple Mold Fresh Kale Shepherds Pie Gravy #2 Cherry Bananas	Vegetable Aspic Broccoli Hollandaise Stuffed Acorn Squash Apple Upside-down Cake	Mushroom Potato Soup Asparagus Crepes Watercress Sauce Peach Cobbler

	Day 1	Day 2	Day 3	Day 4	Day 5	Day 6	Day 7
SNACK							
	Oatmeal Fruit Bars	Halvah on Rice Cakes	Fig Roll Cookies	Nutty Cookies	Banana-Nut Bread	Peanut-Butter Cookies	Carob Chip-Oatmeal Cookies

PLUS ANY HERBAL INFUSION (TEA) SUGGESTED IN THE TEXT ...

	Day 1	Day 2	Day 3	Day 4	Day 5	Day 6	Day 7
LIGHT MEAL							
	Spinach-Miso Soup	V-8® Vegie Soup	Russian Borscht Soup	Blended Salad	Zucchini Soup	Watercress Sprout Salad	Cucumber-Yogurt Soup
	Hommus Sandwich	'Eggless' Salad Sandwich	Tofu Dill Sandwich	Mixed Bean Soup	Grilled 'Cheese' Sandwich	Mushroom Barley Soup	Tofu Burgers
	Pineapple-Strawberry Sherbet	Banana-Strawberry Smoothie	Baked Apples	Fresh Fruit Pie	Carob-Dipped Strawberries	Banana Sherbet	Pineapple-Tapioca Pudding/Pie

Recipe Index

Entrees

Side Dishes

Sauces, Dressings, Miscellaneous

Desserts

Snacks

Breakfasts

BROWN RICE CREAM CEREAL

¼ cup homemade cream of rice (instructions below)
1½ cups water (and pinch of salt, optional)
2 Tbsp. currants
⅓ cup cooked BROWN RICE p. 92

To Prepare the Cream of Rice:
Place 2 cups of uncooked brown rice in a heavy skillet;
heat on medium until lightly toasted, stirring constantly.
Cool and grind in a Vita-Mix® or grain grinder to a fine
powder. Store in a covered jar to use as a cereal or to
thicken soups and sauces.

To Cook the Cereal:
Bring the water and salt to a boil; slowly stir in 3 Tbsp.
of the cream of rice. Lower the heat and simmer for
about 15 minutes, stirring frequently. Add the currants
and brown rice. (A sweetener and/or NUT MILK p. 99 can
be added, if desired.) Serves 1.

BROWN RICE WAFFLES

2 cups cooked BROWN RICE p. 92
2 cups unbleached, whole wheat or brown rice flour
½ tsp. ground cinnamon
½ tsp. ginger
½ tsp. sea salt
½-1 cup chopped pecans

3 cups buttermilk or NUT MILK p. 99
¼ cup maple syrup
½ cup cold pressed oil
2 ripe bananas, mashed
1 tsp. vanilla extract

Combine all the dry ingredients in a large mixing bowl and set aside. In another bowl, combine the wet ingredients (including the bananas) and beat with a whisk until well blended; stir into the dry mixture to form a thick batter. Spoon onto the waffle iron and bake for about 8 minutes each. Makes 8 waffles.

CINNAMON OATMEAL WITH BANANAS AND YOGURT

Prepare the oatmeal as directed for the quantity desired. When the oatmeal is cooked, stir in ⅛ tsp. cinnamon per serving and top with plain yogurt, sliced bananas and 1 tsp. chopped nuts. Add a little fruit juice concentrate or maple syrup for sweetener, if desired.

GRANOLA WITH DRIED FRUIT

Basic Recipe:
¼ cup *each* cold pressed oil and maple syrup
½ tsp. vanilla extract
3 cups oatmeal
¼ tsp. sea salt
½ cup *each* chopped nuts and raisins or chopped dried
    fruit

Dry Ingredients:
Flaked oats, wheat, rye, soy, rice, corn, etc.; assorted seeds; wheat germ and assorted brans; unsweetened protein powder and powdered milk; salt, cinnamon, ginger, lemon peel and other spices; chopped or sliced almonds, cashews, pecans, walnuts or other nuts.

Wet Ingredients:
Cold pressed oil; melted butter or soy margarine; maple syrup; fruit juice concentrates; molasses; rice syrup; barley malt; vanilla extract.

Fruit:
Shredded coconut; raisins; chopped dried dates, apples, figs, apricots, pineapple, prunes, etc.

Use the *Basic Recipe* and add any of the alternative dry and wet ingredients, keeping a ratio of 6 cups dry ingredients to 1 cup wet ingredients and 1 cup fruit. Combine the wet ingredients in one bowl and the dry in another; mix each well. Then combine, mix and roast in a shallow pan at 250°F. for 30 minutes. After roasting, add the dried fruit. The basic recipe makes 4 cups.

For a pie crust, press granola firmly into a pie plate; then fill and bake.

MILLET-SESAME CEREAL WITH BANANAS

1½ cups water
⅓ cup toasted millet-sesame mix (instructions below)
⅛ tsp. sea salt
¼ cup sliced fresh fruit and NUT MILK p. 99

To Prepare the Millet-Sesame Mix:
Place 1 cup raw millet and ¼ cup ground raw sesame seeds in a heavy skillet; stir over medium heat until lightly toasted. Cool and store in a covered jar; cook as needed for breakfast cereal, as a vegetable stuffing or as a grain side dish.

To Cook the Cereal:
In a saucepan, bring the water, millet-sesame mix and salt to a boil. Cover and simmer until the water cooks down and the millet is fluffy, about 20 minutes. Add the sliced fruit and NUT MILK and serve. For additional

sweetener, marinate the fruit in fruit juice concentrate and add along with the milk. Serves 1.

STRAWBERRY-OATMEAL WAFFLES

1 cup fresh or frozen strawberries
½-1 cup chopped pecans
4 cups oatmeal
¼ cup rice flour
1 tsp. *each* sea salt, ginger and cinnamon
4 cups milk, or NUT MILK p. 99
½ cup cold pressed oil
¼ cup sweetener (maple syrup, fruit juice concentrate, etc.)
1 Tbsp. lemon juice
2 tsp. vanilla extract

Set the strawberries and nuts aside. Mix the dry ingredients in a large bowl; stir in the milk. Combine the remaining ingredients and stir into the oatmeal mixture; refrigerate until thick, or prepare and refrigerate the night before. When ready to cook, fold in the strawberries and pecans; spoon the batter onto a preheated waffle iron and cook 7-10 minutes. Serve with STRAWBERRY SAUCE p. 101, maple syrup or plain yogurt. Makes 8 waffles.

WHOLE-GRAIN PANCAKES

1⅓ cups whole-grain flour (rice, buckwheat, millet, rye, corn, etc., or a mixture)
3 tsp. low-sodium baking powder
¼ tsp. sea salt
1 egg or equivalent egg replacer
1 cup NUT MILK p. 99
⅓ cup fruit juice concentrate
1 Tbsp. cold pressed oil

Oil and heat a griddle or heavy skillet while mixing the batter. (The skillet is hot enough when water bounces off.) In a large bowl, mix the flour, baking powder and salt; set aside. In another bowl, combine the wet ingredients and stir into the flour mixture to form a lumpy batter. Pour ¼ cup of the batter onto the griddle for each pancake. Cook on medium heat until tiny bubbles form throughout the pancakes and the edges are slightly dry. Turn and brown on the other side. Serve with CHERRY SAUCE p. 95 or another fruit sauce, compote or jam. Makes 8 pancakes.

Variation:
Fold ½ cup berries or chopped fresh fruit into the batter before cooking.

Soups

CORN CHOWDER

2 Tbsp. butter or soy margarine
1 small onion, chopped
½ cup chopped celery
½ cup dried carrots
2 Tbsp. unbleached wheat or brown rice flour
3 cups vegetable stock
2 cups corn kernels
2 cups cubed potatoes
2 cups NUT MILK p. 99
⅛ tsp. ground nutmeg
2 tsp. herb seasoning salt or 1 tsp. sea salt
Freshly ground pepper to taste

In a large saucepan, sauté the onions, celery and carrots in the butter until tender; add the flour to form a paste and brown lightly. Stir in the stock, corn, and potatoes and simmer until the potatoes are tender, about 20 minutes. Stir in the NUT MILK and seasoning; simmer (*do not boil*) for 10 more minutes, stirring frequently. Adjust the seasoning and garnish with chopped parsley. Serves 4.

CUCUMBER-YOGURT SOUP

4 cucumbers, grated
6 cups plain yogurt
2 cups vegetable stock or water
3 cloves garlic, crushed
2 Tbsp. cider or rice vinegar
1 Tbsp. dried or 2 Tbsp. fresh dill, minced
1 tsp. sea salt
4 Tbsp. cold pressed oil

Combine all the ingredients; mix and chill well before serving. Garnish with a cucumber slice or fresh parsley sprig in each bowl. Serves 6.

MIXED BEAN SOUP

½ cup *each* of six different dried beans (pinto, kidney, navy, lima, garbanzo, Great Northern, adzuki, or black beans)
1½ quarts water for soaking
5 cups vegetable stock or water for cooking
½ cup chopped sweet red peppers
½ cup *each* sliced celery and carrots
1 clove garlic minced, optional
1 bay leaf *and* 1 tsp. dried basil
½ tsp. dried summer savory
¼ tsp. chili powder
2 Tbsp. tamari or ¼ cup liquid soy protein
¼ white wine, optional
1 Tbsp. powdered vegetable broth

½ cup barley
1 cup chopped tomatoes
½ tsp. sea salt, optional
2-3 Tbsp. butter or soy margarine, optional

Rinse the beans well and soak overnight in 1½ quarts of water. When ready to cook, rinse again and drain; cook until tender (about 30 minutes in a pressure cooker). Add the remaining ingredients and simmer until the vegetables are tender. Remove at least 2 cups of the beans and vegetables and purée in a blender or food processor. Return the purée to the soup and add the butter; mix well and serve. Serves 8-10.

MUSHROOM-BARLEY SOUP

1 medium onion, chopped
2-3 stalks celery, cut into 1-inch pieces
3 carrots, cut into 1-inch pieces
1 lb. mushrooms, sliced
1 cup barley
2½ quarts vegetable stock or water
Sea salt or tamari and freshly ground pepper to taste
Fresh parsley, chopped

In a covered pot, steam the celery, carrots and ⅓ of the mushrooms until tender; then purée in a food processor, adding vegetable stock as needed. Sauté the onion and the rest of the mushrooms until tender. Place the vegetable purée, sautéed mixture and the rest of the stock in a large pot; add the barley and season to taste. Cook on low heat about 1½ hours (the longer it cooks, the better it tastes and the thicker it gets). Garnish with chopped parsley and serve. Purée leftovers and use as a gravy. Serves 8.

MUSHROOM-POTATO SOUP

½ lb. mushrooms, sliced
½ cup sliced onion
½ cup sliced celery
2 Tbsp. butter or soy margarine
1 lb. potatoes, thinly sliced
1 bay leaf
1 tsp. dried parsley
1 large carrot, sliced
1 tsp. powdered vegetable broth
3 cups vegetable stock
Sea salt and freshly ground pepper to taste
LOW-FAT 'SOUR CREAM' p. 97, optional

Set the sour cream aside. In a large pot, sauté the mushrooms, onion and celery in the butter until tender. Add the remaining ingredients; simmer for 20 minutes. Season to taste; serve with a spoonful of sour cream in each bowl. Serves 4.

RUSSIAN BORSCHT

1 lb. fresh beetroots
4 cups vegetable stock
4 medium potatoes, sliced
1 medium onion, sliced
2 small carrots, sliced
2 stalks celery, sliced
1 bay leaf
1 large ripe tomato, peeled and wedged
Sea salt and freshly ground pepper to taste
LOW-FAT 'SOUR CREAM' p. 97, optional

Peel and thinly slice the beets; place with the vegetable stock in a large soup pot. Bring to a boil; reduce the heat and simmer for 15 minutes. Add the potatoes, onions, carrots, celery and bay leaf (add more vegetable stock, if necessary). Cook for 15 more minutes; add the tomatoes and seasonings. Cook until all the vegetables are tender. Remove the bay leaf and serve hot with a spoonful of 'sour cream' in each bowl. Serves 4-6.

SPINACH-MISO SOUP

1 Tbsp. sesame oil (toasted, if available)
4 green onions, sliced
¼ lb. tofu, cut in ½-inch cubes
5 cups water
1 cup chopped spinach (fresh or frozen)
1 carrot, sliced
¼ cup miso

In a soup pot, sauté the green onions and tofu cubes in the sesame oil. Add the water, spinach and carrots; bring to a boil. Reduce the heat and cover. Simmer until the vegetables are just tender, 20-30 minutes. Remove from the heat. Dissolve the miso in about ¼ cup of the soup broth and stir into the soup; cover and set aside for about 5 minutes before serving. Serves 4.

V-8® VEGIE SOUP

48-oz. can V-8® Juice or a mixed vegetable juice
1 small onion, chopped
2 carrots, sliced
2 stalks celery, sliced
6 new potatoes, diced
Handful of cauliflowerettes, green beans, shredded cabbage and/or any other raw or leftover vegetables
⅛ tsp. basil
¼ tsp. parsley
⅛ tsp. garlic powder or 1 crushed garlic clove
Water to cover vegetables

Place all ingredients in a large pot and simmer until the

vegetables are tender, about 30 minutes. Serve with a garnish of chopped, fresh parsley. Serves 6-8.

ZUCCHINI SOUP

6 small zucchini, cut into chunks
1 large onion, thinly sliced
1 tsp. curry powder
½ tsp. ground ginger
½ tsp. dry mustard
1 tsp. powdered vegetable broth
3 cups vegetable stock
3 Tbsp. uncooked brown rice
1½ cups milk or NUT MILK p. 99
Sea salt and freshly ground pepper to taste
Minced chives for garnish

Combine the zucchini, onion, curry powder, ginger, mustard and powdered vegetable broth in a saucepan; add the vegetable stock and rice and bring to a boil. Cover and simmer for 45 minutes. Transfer the mixture to a blender or food processor and purée; add the milk and season to taste. Reheat (do not boil); serve hot or cold. Garnish with minced chives. Serves 6.

Salads

BLENDED SALAD

1 carrot
1 stalk celery
½ fresh beet
½ cucumber
Small bunch parsley
10 romaine lettuce leaves
1 tomato

Any other favorite vegetables
MISO DRESSING p. 98

In a food processor, separately prepare the following: grate the carrot and beet; chop the firm vegetables together (celery, cucumber, parsley); chop the lettuce, a few leaves at a time, then the tomato. Toss all the vegetables together. Add MISO DRESSING, toss again and top with garbanzo or other beans, nuts, seeds, grated cheese, etc. Serves 4.

CARROT-RAISIN SALAD

4 medium carrots, grated
½ cup raisins
½ cup shredded unsweetened coconut
2 Tbsp. lemon juice
¼ cup TOFU MAYONNAISE p. 102
1 tsp. celery seeds, optional
2 Tbsp. apple juice concentrate, optional

Combine all the ingredients in a large bowl and toss well. Chill and serve on a bed of lettuce leaves. Serves 6-8.

STUFFED BEETS

8 fresh medium-sized beets
2 Tbsp. *each* oil and lemon juice or wine vinegar
1 tsp. Dijon-style mustard
Sea salt and pepper to taste
½ cup sour cream or LOW-FAT 'SOUR CREAM' p. 97
1½ Tbsp. prepared horseradish, drained
½ tsp. Dijon-style mustard

Wash the beets well and steam until tender. Cool, peel and level off the bottom of the beets to stand up straight. Scoop out the center of each beet, leaving a shell about ¼-inch thick. Chop the beet centers finely to use in the stuffing. Mix the oil, lemon, 1 tsp. mustard, salt and pepper together and marinate the beets in this dressing for about 1 hour, turning frequently. Meanwhile, combine the sour cream, horseradish, ½ tsp. mustard and chopped beet centers; mix well and season to taste. Just before serving, drain the beets; fill the centers with the sour cream mixture. Serve 2 stuffed beets on a bed of lettuce for each person. Serves 4.

TANGY APPLE MOLD

½ cup agar-agar flakes
2 cups HOMEMADE APPLESAUCE p. 97
1 cup carbonated water
1 tsp. grated orange peel
¼ cup orange juice concentrate
1 cup chopped apple
¼ cup chopped walnuts
2 Tbsp. *each* fresh lemon juice and sweetener
TOFU MAYONNAISE p. 102
Lettuce leaves and fresh watercress

In a saucepan, heat the applesauce and agar-agar; simmer for 5 minutes. Remove from the heat and cool. Stir in the carbonated water, orange juice and peel; chill until partially set. Toss the chopped apple and walnuts in the lemon juice and sweetener; add to the applesauce mixture and turn into a 4- or 5-cup ring mold. Chill until firmly set; unmold on lettuce leaves. Top with TOFU MAYONNAISE and garnish with watercress. Serves 6-8.

VEGETABLE ASPIC

2 Tbsp. oil
½ cup chopped onion
1 28-oz. can peeled, crushed tomatoes
1 bay leaf and ¼ tsp. paprika
1 clove of garlic, minced or ⅛ tsp. garlic powder

½ cup agar-agar flakes
2 Tbsp. tamari
1 Tbsp. cider or rice vinegar
Juice and grated peel from ½ lemon
½ cup grated carrot and radish
½ cup chopped celery
½ cup chopped cucumber, olives and/or any other
  vegetable
Sea salt and pepper to taste
Small bunch of watercress

In a large skillet, sauté the onions in the oil until
tender. Add the tomatoes, bay leaf, garlic and paprika;
cook gently for 10 minutes. Add the agar-agar and cook
for 5 more minutes, stirring continuously. Add the
tamari, vinegar, lemon peel and juice and vegetables;
season to taste. Pour into a large oiled ring mold and
chill for several hours. When ready to serve, turn the
aspic onto a bed of lettuce, and garnish with fresh
watercress. Serve with TOFU MAYONNAISE p. 102, or MISO
DRESSING p. 98. Serves 8.

WATERCRESS-STRINGBEAN SALAD

1 medium potato, cooked and diced
1 lb. fresh string beans, cooked and cut in 1-inch pieces
1 large bunch watercress, trimmed and chopped
½ medium red onion, thinly sliced
1 medium cucumber, thinly sliced
1 cup sliced mushrooms
1 cup 'SOUR CREAM' DRESSING p. 101
Sea salt and pepper to taste

Combine all the vegetables in a large bowl. Add the
'SOUR CREAM' DRESSING; toss and season to taste. Serve
on a bed of romaine lettuce. Serves 6-8.

WATERCRESS-SPROUT SALAD

1 cup watercress
4 romaine lettuce leaves
1 cup alfalfa sprouts
¼ cup ground toasted sesame seeds
¼ cup grated carrots
MISO DRESSING p. 98

Remove the thick stems from the watercress. Tear or cut the lettuce into bite-sized pieces. Combine all the ingredients and toss gently until well coated with the MISO DRESSING or dressing of choice. Serves 4.

Entrees

ASPARAGUS CREPES

24 fresh asparagus spears
WATERCRESS SAUCE p. 102
8 WHOLE WHEAT CREPES (below)

To prepare the asparagus for cooking: hold the stem and the tip ends between the fingertips of each hand. Bend the asparagus until it breaks. Discard the stem ends and steam the tips until tender-crisp. Prepare the WATER-CRESS SAUCE and the WHOLE WHEAT CREPES. Place 3 asparagus spears in the center of each crepe and spoon on 2 Tbsp. of the WATERCRESS SAUCE. Roll the crepes and arrange them, side by side, in a baking dish; top with the remaining sauce and bake in a preheated oven at 400°F. for about 10 minutes. Serve immediately. Serves 4.

WHOLE WHEAT CREPES

2 eggs or equivalent egg replacer

½ tsp. sea salt
1 cup whole wheat flour
1¼ cups milk or NUT MILK p. 99
Cold pressed oil for frying

Beat the eggs or egg replacer and salt together; stir in the flour. Add the milk and beat to a thin, smooth batter (add extra milk if necessary). Set aside for about 20 minutes. Meanwhile, heat a crepe pan or a 7-inch, heavy-bottomed skillet on medium heat. When hot, brush it with oil and pour in 2 Tbsp. of the batter. Tilt the pan quickly so that the batter spreads evenly over the bottom of the skillet. When the batter is set and the surface has turned dull, turn it over gently and cook the other side. Remove the crepe from the pan; place it on a lightly buttered plate on top of a pan of boiling water (to keep it warm and moist while cooking the rest). Repeat the process for each crepe, stacking them on top of each other, until the batter is used.

Fill the crepes with vegetables or fruit and an accompanying sauce; serve immediately. (The cooked crepes may be refrigerated or individually wrapped and frozen to fill and serve later.) Serves 4.

BROCCOLI-CAULIFLOWER CASSEROLE

BROWN RICE crust p. 92
TOFU 'RICOTTA CHEESE' p. 102
1 head *each* broccoli and cauliflower
4 Tbsp. butter or soy margarine
3 Tbsp. liquid soy protein or tamari
2 Tbsp. powdered vegetable broth
½ tsp. sea salt and freshly ground pepper to taste
¼ cup minced parsley

Oil a large baking dish. Press BROWN RICE into a crust 1-inch thick and set aside. Prepare the TOFU

'RICOTTA CHEESE' and set aside. Wash the cauliflower and broccoli and cut into bite-sized pieces; steam lightly. In a large skillet, melt the butter; add the seasonings and cauliflower and broccoli pieces and sauté for 5 minutes, stirring frequently. Add the 'cheese' and mix well. Pour into the crust and sprinkle with minced parsley. Bake in a preheated oven at 350°F. for 20 minutes. Serves 8.

'EGGLESS' SALAD SANDWICH

1 lb. tofu
3 Tbsp. Dijon-style mustard
1 tsp. curry powder
1 tsp. dried or 2 tsp. fresh basil
$\frac{1}{3}$ cup TOFU MAYONNAISE p. 102
2-3 green onions, chopped
2-3 stalks celery, chopped
$\frac{1}{4}$ cup chopped fresh parsley
Herb seasoning salt, optional
Freshly ground pepper to taste

In a large bowl, crumble the tofu; add the remaining ingredients and mix well. Serve in a pita bread sandwich with lettuce and tomato (or as a tomato stuffing or a spread for crackers). Serves 4.

HOMMUS SANDWICH

3 cups cooked garbanzo beans (chickpeas)
2 cloves garlic, minced
$\frac{1}{3}$ cup fresh lemon juice
1 tsp. sea salt or to taste
$\frac{1}{2}$ cup tahini (sesame seed paste)
2 Tbsp. cold pressed oil
$\frac{1}{3}$ cup chopped fresh parsley

½ cup plain yogurt, optional
Alfalfa sprouts, lettuce and sliced tomatoes

Blend all the ingredients in a food processor or blender until smooth and creamy. Serve as a filling for pita bread with lettuce, tomato and sprouts (or as a dip for cut fresh vegetables). Makes 4 cups.

GRILLED 'CHEESE' SANDWICH

8 slices whole-grain bread, toasted
1 lb. tofu (firm)
⅓ cup white miso
½ tsp. toasted sesame oil
2 Tbsp. *each* cold pressed oil and tahini
1 tsp. minced fresh parsley

Place the toast on a cookie sheet and set aside. Slice the tofu into at least 8 thin slices as wide as the block; dry each slice and set aside. Combine the remaining ingredients and mix well. Spread a little of the mixture on each piece of toast and cover with a tofu slice, then top with the remaining mixture. Broil until golden brown, about 10 minutes. Serves 8.

LENTIL-VEGIE LOAF

½ cup chopped onion
2 stalks celery, chopped
1 small carrot, chopped
2 small tomatoes, chopped
2 cups cooked BROWN RICE p. 92
1½ cups bread crumbs (10 slices)
½ cup chopped walnuts
2 cups cooked lentils
¼ cup chopped green olives
1 tsp. sea salt *and* 2 tsp. powdered vegetable broth
2 eggs or equivalent egg replacer

In a large skillet, sauté the chopped vegetables until tender. Add the remaining ingredients and mix well. Form into a loaf and bake in an oiled loaf pan for about 45 minutes at 350°F. or form into burgers and bake or fry. Serve with rice and gravy. Serves 6-8.

SHEPHERDS PIE

1 uncooked pie crust
6 medium potatoes, diced
2 carrots, diced
2 cups cooked Great Northern beans
½-1 cup GRAVY I or II pp. 99, 100
2 cups cooked field peas or black-eyed peas
1 cup cooked lima beans
½ tsp. basil
¼ tsp. marjoram
¼ cup tamari or ⅓ cup liquid soy protein
A little milk, soy milk or NUT MILK p. 99
2 Tbsp. butter or soy margarine
Sea salt and pepper to taste

Prepare 1 crust and set aside, unbaked. Steam the diced potatoes and carrots, placing the carrots over to one side, so that some potatoes can later be removed to mash for the topping. Meanwhile, combine the Great Northern beans and gravy in a food processor or blender; process until smooth. Combine the bean mixture in a large bowl with the field peas, lima beans, basil, marjoram and tamari; mix well.

When the potatoes and carrots are tender, remove 2½ cups of potatoes and blend with a little milk, butter, salt and pepper to make a mashed potato topping; set aside. Gently fold the remaining potatoes and carrots into the bean mixture and pour into the pie crust. Spread the mashed potatoes over the top and bake in a preheated oven at 350°F. for about 45 minutes, until the crust and topping are lightly browned. (This dish can be prepared hours ahead and baked just before serving.) Serves 6-8.

STUFFED ACORN SQUASH

3 acorn squash
1 lb. tofu
¾ cup brown rice flour
½ tsp. sea salt and pepper to taste
1 medium onion, or 6-8 green onions, chopped
1 celery stalk, sliced
1 carrot, grated
⅓ cup fresh parsley, chopped
1 cup cooked MILLET p. 93
½ cup chopped sesame or sunflower seeds
½ cup fresh or canned hot taco sauce

Stuffing:
In a large bowl, crumble the tofu. Add the rice flour, salt and pepper and toss until the tofu is well coated with flour. Place the mixture in a heated frying pan with enough oil to cover the bottom. Fry on medium-high heat for about 45 minutes, until the tofu is very crisp and golden brown; stir frequently. Add the onions and celery and carrots; sauté until tender. Add the parsley, millet, seeds and hot sauce and mix well.

Squash:
Wash and cut the acorn squash in half; remove the seeds and place in a large steamer. Steam until almost done but still firm; remove from the heat, uncover, and set aside. Spoon the stuffing into the center of each squash half; place in a large baking dish or pan with a little water in the bottom. Bake at 350°F. for about 30 minutes or until the squash is soft. Garnish with tomato wedges and parsley sprigs. Serves 6.

TOFU BURGERS

2 lb. tofu
1 medium onion, chopped
½ lb. carrots, grated
½-1 cup fresh or canned hot taco sauce
¼ tsp. basil
½-1 tsp. sea salt
1 cup finely chopped roasted peanuts
¼ cup chopped fresh parsley
1 egg or equivalent egg replacer
1 cup brown rice flour

In a large mixing bowl, crumble the tofu with your fingers and set aside. Sauté the onions in a little oil and add to the tofu. Add the remaining ingredients and mix well. Form into patties and fry until browned and crisp on both sides, or bake at 350°F. until firm and browned, about 30 minutes. Serve on pita bread with sliced vegetables or with rice, vegetables and gravy. (Uneaten burgers may be frozen and reheated when needed.) Makes about 2 dozen burgers.

TOFU CROQUETTES

3 cups cooked BROWN RICE p. 92
2 lb. tofu, crumbled
½ cup rice flour
2 Tbsp. butter or soy margarine
1 cup chopped celery
½ cup chopped onion
¼ cup chopped fresh parsley
¼ cup tamari
3 eggs or equivalent egg replacer
2 tsp. powdered vegetable broth
1-2 tsp. herb seasoning salt or sea salt
¼ tsp. garlic powder
1 8-oz. can water chestnuts, chopped

½ cup peanut butter
½ cup chopped walnuts
Enough gravy to moisten
Buttermilk, optional

In a large mixing bowl, combine the rice, tofu, and flour and set aside. Sauté the celery and onions in the butter until tender. Add the remaining ingredients and mix well. Combine with the rice-tofu mixture and work with your hands until well mixed. Form into patties or cone-shaped croquettes and place on an oiled baking sheet; coat the tops with buttermilk and bake in a preheated oven at 375°F. for about 30 minutes. Serve with gravy. Makes about 2 dozen patties.

TOFU-DILL SANDWICH

1 lb. tofu
2 Tbsp. lemon juice
2 Tbsp. cold pressed oil
½ tsp. sea salt
½-1 tsp. dill weed or seeds
2 Tbsp. chopped fresh parsley
Pinch of garlic powder

Blend the tofu with the remaining ingredients in a food processor or blender until smooth and creamy. Or crumble the tofu finely and mix well with the remaining ingredients for a different texture. (Note: to freshen older tofu, drop into boiling water for 2-3 minutes, cool and use in recipe.) Serve chilled as a sandwich spread with sliced tomato, lettuce and sprouts. Makes 2 cups.

TOFU-MUSHROOM STROGANOFF

2 lb. tofu
1 lb. fresh mushrooms
1 Tbsp. butter

1 Tbsp. wine of choice
½ cup tamari
½ tsp. garlic powder
2 tsp. dried chives
¼ cup wine of choice
1 tsp. powdered vegetable broth
½ cup water
Several good turns freshly ground pepper
1 medium onion, thinly sliced
½ cup tomato purée
2 Tbsp. ROUX p. 100
1 cup sour cream
1 pkg. Jerusalem artichoke or rice noodles

Slice the tofu into thin strips (about ¼" x ¾" x 3"). Fry the tofu strips on both sides in a little oil until golden brown and crisp. (2 skillets save time.) Drain on paper towels and set aside.

Wipe the mushrooms clean with a damp cloth (don't soak as they absorb too much water); slice in half. In a large skillet or saucepan, melt the butter and add 1 Tbsp. of wine and the mushrooms; cover and sauté for about 5 minutes. (Start the noodles cooking.)

Add the tamari, garlic powder, chives, wine, powdered broth, water, pepper and onions to the saucepan; bring to a boil. Reduce the heat and simmer about 5 minutes. Add the tomato purée and whisk in the ROUX to thicken. Add the tofu; simmer to blend the flavors, about 5 minutes. Remove from the heat; add the sour cream and serve over a bed of hot noodles. Serves 6.

Side Dishes

BROCCOLI HOLLANDAISE

1 large head broccoli

'HOLLANDAISE' SAUCE p. 96

Break or cut the broccoli into bite-sized pieces and place in steamer basket in a large pot; add water to cover bottom of pot (about 1-inch high or more, if you want to save the stock for later). Bring to a boil, cover, reduce the heat and simmer until the broccoli is tender-crisp. Meanwhile, prepare the 'HOLLANDAISE' SAUCE. Place the steamed broccoli in a heated serving dish, cover with the sauce, and serve. Serves 6-8.

BROWN RICE

2 cups brown rice
4 cups water

Rinse the brown rice well; drain and set aside. Bring the water to a boil in a large saucepan. Add the rice; stir once (do not stir again or it will become sticky). Cover, reduce the heat and simmer for 55 minutes (until the water is absorbed). Turn off the heat and let the cooked rice sit on the warm burner until ready to serve. Makes about 5 cups.

(Note: the amount of water and length of cooking time may vary according to the type of cooking vessels or source of heat used. Adjust accordingly.)

Variations:
1. Substitute tomato juice, fruit juice or vegetable bouillon for the water.
2. Top hot cooked rice with butter and chopped parsley, chives or celery seeds.
3. Add ½ cup washed millet or kasha and 1 more cup water to the rice and cook together.
4. To make a crust for vegetable pies, press cooked rice firmly into the bottom and sides of an oiled pie plate.

ENDIVE POTATOES

8 cups chopped new potatoes (unpeeled)
1 cup chopped onion
6 Tbsp. butter or soy margarine
4 cups chopped fresh Belgian endive
¼ cup tamari

Wash the potatoes well and steam or boil until tender. Sauté the onions and endive in the butter until tender and add with the tamari to the potatoes (still hot). Mash everything together and serve as a side dish. Serves 6.

FRESH STEAMED KALE

4 lb. fresh kale or other greens, washed and chopped
¼ cup butter or soy margarine
3 Tbsp. powdered vegetable broth
1 tsp. herb seasoning salt or ½ tsp. sea salt
1-2 Tbsp. lemon juice

Steam the kale until tender, about 15 minutes. Add the remaining ingredients, mix well and place in a heated serving bowl. (If fresh greens are not available, frozen may be substituted.) Serves 6.

MILLET

1½ cups millet
3 cups water
1 tsp. powdered vegetable broth, optional

Wash the millet well; drain and set aside. Bring the water to a boil; add the millet and powdered broth, stir once and cover. (Do not stir while cooking or it will become sticky.) Simmer until the water is absorbed, about 20 minutes. Serve plain with butter or gravy, or mixed with sautéed green onions, parsley, green peas and carrots. Makes about 3½ cups.

SAUTÉED PARSNIPS AND CARROTS

½ lb. carrots, cut into julienne strips
½ lb. parsnips, cut into julienne strips
¼ cup plain yogurt
1 Tbsp. fresh parsley, minced
2 tsp. minced fresh dill or 1 tsp. dried dill
2 Tbsp. butter or soy margarine (skip this step if serving cold as a salad)
Sea salt and freshly ground pepper to taste

Steam the carrots for about 5 minutes; add the parsnips and steam until tender. Combine the remaining ingredients and set aside. When the vegetables are cooked, drain and stir in the yogurt mixture. Serve hot or cold. Serves 4.

Sauces, Dressings, Miscellaneous

ALMOND CREAM

½ cup blanched almonds
½ cup water
2 pitted dates or dried figs
¼ tsp. orange or apple juice concentrate
Pinch of sea salt

In a food processor or blender, chop the almonds to a fine powder; add the remaining ingredients and process until smooth. Serve in place of dairy cream, over fruit, pies or grains. Makes 1 cup.

APPLE SAUCE

2 cups apple juice
2 Tbsp. cornstarch, potato starch or arrowroot
2 Tbsp. butter or soy margarine

½ tsp. vanilla extract
Pinch of cinnamon, optional

In a small saucepan, bring 1¾ cups of the apple juice to a boil. Dissolve the potato starch or arrowroot in the remaining ¼ cup of apple juice and add to the boiling juice, stirring continuously until thickened. Remove from the heat, and stir in the butter and vanilla extract. Serve warm, over APPLE UPSIDE-DOWN CAKE p. 103, or any breakfast pancake, waffle, muffin or biscuit. Makes about 2 cups.

CASHEW CREAM

½ cup cashews
½ cup water
1 Tbsp. sweetener (maple syrup, apple juice concentrate, rice syrup, etc.)
¼ tsp. vanilla extract
Pinch of sea salt, optional

In a food processor or blender, chop the cashews to a fine powder; add the remaining ingredients and process until smooth. Serve as you would dairy cream, over fruit, pies or grains. Makes 1 cup.

CHERRY SAUCE

2 cups fresh pitted cherries or 1 16-oz. can unsweetened sour cherries
½ cup frozen apple juice concentrate
2 Tbsp. black cherry concentrate
2 Tbsp. flour or arrowroot
¼ cup apple juice

Rinse and drain the cherries; purée in a food processor with the apple and black cherry concentrates. Transfer the purée to a saucepan and bring to a boil; reduce the heat. Dissolve the flour or arrowroot in the apple juice and add it to the purée, stirring continuously until the mixture thickens. Serve hot or cold on pancakes and waffles, as a spread for muffins or biscuits. Makes about 2 cups.

FIG LASSI

⅓ cup syrup from soaked dried figs
⅔ cup buttermilk
Ice chips

Fill a screw-top jar with dried figs and cover with water. Refrigerate for at least 24 hours before serving. Shake the jar occasionally to mix the liquid. The longer the figs soak, the thicker and sweeter the syrup becomes.

Combine the buttermilk with the fig syrup and stir. Add ice chips and garnish with a sprig of fresh mint. Serves 1.

FRENCH LEMON DRESSING

½ cup cold pressed olive oil
⅓ cup fresh lemon juice
1 tsp. grated lemon peel
1 Tbsp. cider or rice vinegar
1 tsp. dry mustard
1 Tbsp. apple juice concentrate
¼ tsp. herb seasoning salt or sea salt
⅛ tsp. ground white pepper

Combine all the ingredients in a screw-top jar; shake well and chill. Shake again before serving over salad greens. Makes 1 cup.

'HOLLANDAISE' SAUCE

3 Tbsp. butter or soy margarine
3 Tbsp. rice flour

1½ cups cashew milk (see NUT MILK p. 99)
⅓ cup lemon juice
⅛ tsp. cayenne pepper (more to taste)
Sea salt to taste

Melt the butter in a medium-sized saucepan on low heat.
Add the flour and mix well. Slowly add the cashew milk,
stirring until the mixture is quite thick and creamy.
Remove from the heat. Add the lemon juice, cayenne
pepper and salt; mix well. Serve over steamed vegetables
or crepes. Makes about 1¾ cups.

HOMEMADE APPLESAUCE

6 baking apples
½ cup raisins
½ cup apple juice
1 tsp. cinnamon
A squeeze of fresh lemon juice

Core and chop the apples; place in large saucepan with
the remaining ingredients. Bring to a boil and simmer
until well done. Serve with toast, pancakes or waffles or
as a main meal side dish. Makes about 3 cups.

LOW-FAT 'SOUR CREAM'

½ cup skim milk
½ cup farmer's, ricotta or low-fat cottage cheese

In a blender or food processor, blend the cheese and milk
to the desired consistency. Serve whenever sour cream
would be appropriate. Makes 1 cup.

M(APPLE) SYRUP

3 cups apple juice
1 cup maple syrup
½ cup apple juice concentrate

3 Tbsp. agar-agar
Pinch of sea salt
½ tsp. vanilla extract

Combine all the ingredients except the vanilla in a saucepan and bring to the boil. Reduce the heat and simmer for 5 minutes, stirring continuously. Remove from the heat; stir in the vanilla and chill. When set, *shake well* or whisk to help the syrup pour evenly. Serve over waffles, pancakes or puddings. Makes 4½ cups.

MISO DRESSING

⅓ cup miso
⅓ cup tahini
¼ cup lemon juice
¾-1 cup vegetable stock
1 clove garlic, minced or ¼ tsp. garlic powder

Whisk all the ingredients together until smooth and chill well before serving. Makes 1¼ cups.

MISO GRAVY

2 Tbsp. butter or soy margarine
3 Tbsp. rice flour
3 cups vegetable stock
¼ tsp. dried or ½ tsp. chopped fresh basil
⅛ tsp. dried or ¼ tsp. chopped fresh marjoram
¼ cup miso

Melt the butter in a small saucepan; stir in the flour to make a paste. Add the vegetable stock and herbs, stirring continuously, until thickened; remove from the heat. Dissolve the miso in a small amount of the gravy; then return to the soup and serve. Makes 3 cups.

NUT BUTTER

2 cups raw or lightly toasted nuts (cashews, blanched
  almonds, pecans or peanuts)
Sea salt to taste, optional

Chop the nuts in a food processor or grinder to the
desired consistency. (The longer the processing, the more
oil is released.) Add salt if desired and blend again.
Makes about 1½ cups.

NUT MILK

1 cup nuts (blanched almonds, cashews, pecans, etc.)
3 cups water

Chop the nuts in a blender or food processor until finely
powdered; add the water and blend for 3 minutes. Strain,
if desired, and reserve the nut pulp for cereal or baking.
Mix well and serve hot or cold. Makes 1 quart.

Note: when serving NUT MILK as a beverage or with
cereal, etc., add:

  2 tsp. sweetener (barley malt, carob, rice syrup,
    maple syrup, apple juice concentrate)
  1 tsp. vanilla extract

GRAVY I

2 Tbsp. butter or soy margarine
½ cup brown rice flour
3 cups vegetable stock or water
¼ cup tamari or liquid soy protein
1 Tbsp. wine
1 tsp. powdered vegetable broth
Sprinkle of summer savory
½-1 tsp. herb seasoning salt and pepper to taste
1-2 Tbsp. lemon juice

Melt the butter in a small saucepan; stir in the flour to form a paste. Add the remaining ingredients (except for the lemon juice), stirring continuously, until thickened. Add the lemon juice; season to taste. Serve with any loaf/burger recipes. Makes 3 cups.

GRAVY II

¼ cup finely chopped onion
2 Tbsp. cold pressed oil
2 peeled tomatoes, coarsely chopped
2 cups vegetable stock
¼ cup tamari
Pinch of dried thyme
1 bay leaf
¼ cup red wine
1 tsp. powdered vegetable broth
Freshly ground pepper to taste
1 Tbsp. flour or arrowroot

Sauté the onion in the oil until golden brown; add the tomatoes and cook, stirring continuously until the liquid has evaporated. Add 1½ cups of the vegetable stock and the herbs and seasonings; simmer for about 20 minutes, stirring occasionally. Remove the bay leaf and purée the gravy in a food processor or blender; reheat. Dissolve the flour in the remaining vegetable stock and add to the tomatoes, stirring continuously until thickened. Serve with any loaf or burger recipes. Makes about 2 cups.

ROUX

½ cup unsalted butter
1 Tbsp. cold pressed oil
1 cup flour (unbleached, whole wheat, rice flour, etc.)

Melt the butter in a small saucepan; add the oil (to

keep the butter from burning) and stir in the flour. Cook on low heat for a few minutes, stirring continuously, until thickened. Cool and roll into one-tablespoon balls for easy use. Can be kept refrigerated in a covered container for a couple of months. Use in TOFU-MUSHROOM STROGANOFF p. 90 or as needed to thicken soups and sauces. Makes 1½ cups.

'SOUR CREAM' DRESSING

1 cup TOFU MAYONNAISE p. 102
¼ cup fresh lemon juice
2 tsp. cider or rice vinegar
½-1 tsp. sea salt
1 tsp. dried or 2-3 tsp. fresh dill weed
Freshly ground pepper to taste
3 Tbsp. sweetener (rice syrup or apple juice concentrate), optional

Whisk all ingredients together until completely blended. Chill and serve on WATERCRESS – STRING-BEAN SALAD p. 82 or other salads. Makes about 1½ cups.

STRAWBERRY SAUCE

½ cup strawberry concentrate
2 Tbsp. maple syrup
2 cups sliced strawberries
2 Tbsp. potato starch, flour or arrowroot
¼ cup apple juice

Place the strawberry concentrate, maple syrup and strawberries in a small saucepan; bring to a boil. Dissolve the thickener in the apple juice and add to the strawberries. Reduce the heat and stir continuously until the sauce has thickened. Serve over pancakes, waffles or biscuits. Makes about 2 cups.

TOFU MAYONNAISE

1 lb. tofu
⅓ cup cold pressed oil
⅓ cup lemon juice
½ tsp. onion powder
½ tsp. dry mustard
1 tsp. herb seasoning salt or ½ tsp. sea salt
⅛ tsp. garlic powder or to taste
1 tsp. apple juice concentrate
(Italian herbs to taste for variety)

Blend the tofu in a food processor until smooth; add the oil, lemon juice and seasonings and blend. Add more oil or lemon juice or a little water to adjust the consistency. Makes about 2½ cups.

TOFU 'RICOTTA CHEESE'

1 lb. tofu
2 Tbsp. cold pressed oil
¼ cup lemon juice
¼ tsp. basil
1 tsp. Italian herbs
⅛ tsp. garlic powder or 1 small clove garlic
3 green onions, chopped or ¼ tsp. onion powder
2 tsp. chopped fresh or 1 tsp. dried parsley
1 tsp. powdered vegetable broth
½ tsp. sea salt or to taste

Blend the tofu in a food processor until creamy or crumble finely with your fingers. Add the oil, lemon juice, herbs, green onions and salt; mix well. Use in lasagna, manicotti, casseroles, etc. Makes about 2½ cups.

WATERCRESS SAUCE

1 cup chopped watercress

¼ cup cold pressed olive oil
2 tsp. Dijon-style mustard
2 Tbsp. lemon juice, cider or rice vinegar
1 cup LOW-FAT 'SOUR CREAM' p. 97
Sea salt and pepper to taste

Blend all the ingredients in a food processor or blender until smooth. Serve over ASPARAGUS CREPES p. 83 or grains and salads. Makes 1½ cups.

Desserts

APPLE UPSIDE-DOWN CAKE

2 cups chopped apples
1 heaped tsp. cinnamon
½ cup raisins
½ cup chopped nuts
1 egg or equivalent egg replacer
2 Tbsp. butter or soy margarine
2 Tbsp. apple juice concentrate
2 Tbsp. maple syrup
½ cup buttermilk or NUT MILK p. 99
1 Tbsp. cider or rice vinegar
1 tsp. baking soda
1¼ cups unbleached wheat flour

Preheat the oven to 350°F. Mix the chopped apples, raisins, nuts and cinnamon together and place in the bottom of an oiled 8-inch square pan. Melt the butter and combine with the other wet ingredients; set aside. Sift the flour and baking soda together. Add the wet ingredients and mix well; pour over the apple mixture and bake for 30 minutes. Cool slightly and flip over onto a plate, apple side up. Pour warm APPLE SAUCE p. 94 on top and serve. Serves 8.

BAKED APPLES

4 baking apples
2 Tbsp. butter or soy margarine
1 tsp. cinnamon
4 dried figs, chopped
8 dried apricots, chopped
½ cup raisins
¼ cup apple juice concentrate
¼ cup chopped walnuts

Wash and core the apples, leaving ½ inch at the bottom; set aside. Combine the remaining ingredients and mix well. Spoon the stuffing into the cored apples and bake at 350°F. until tender, about 30 minutes. Serves 4.

BANANA SHERBET

Peel overripe bananas (allow 1 banana per serving) and freeze overnight in a plastic bag. Chop into ½-inch pieces and blend in a food processor or blender until creamy. Add a little apple juice, if needed, to help blend. Serve with a fresh strawberry, sprig of mint, slice of orange or nuts as a garnish.

BANANA-STRAWBERRY SMOOTHIE

½ banana, frozen
3 strawberries, frozen
½ cup apple juice

In a blender or food processor, place the suggested fruit combination (or experiment with your own); add 1 Tbsp. unsweetened protein powder, if desired, and blend until smooth. Add crushed ice and serve. Makes 1 cup.

CAROB-DIPPED STRAWBERRIES

Carob Coating:
¼ cup butter or soy margarine
¼ cup maple syrup
6 Tbsp. carob powder
¼ cup dairy, soy or NUT MILK p. 99
½ tsp. vanilla extract
A pinch of sea salt

Fruit:
2 pints fresh strawberries or other fruit of choice
1 cup finely chopped pecans

Melt the butter in a small saucepan. Add the maple syrup, carob powder, milk and salt; mix well and simmer for about 5 minutes, stirring continuously. Add the vanilla and stir well; set aside to cool. Dip each piece of fruit into the cooled carob mixture until well coated; roll the strawberries in the pecans. Place on wax paper or a buttered platter to set. If the kitchen is too warm for the carob to set properly, place in the refrigerator or freezer until ready to serve as a snack or dessert. Serves 8.

CHERRY BANANAS

1 Tbsp. butter or soy margarine
3 Tbsp. black cherry concentrate
4 medium bananas, cut diagonally into ½-inch
  chunks
1 cup pitted cherries
½ cup seltzer water
¼ cup black cherry concentrate
¼ tsp. ground cinnamon
2 Tbsp. arrowroot

Melt the butter in a saucepan; add the 3 Tbsp. black

cherry concentrate, the bananas and the cherries and stir until well coated. Remove and set aside. Combine the remaining ingredients in the saucepan and bring to a boil; reduce the heat and simmer for 5 minutes, stirring continuously. Pour over the bananas and cherries and serve warm or chilled. Serves 6.

FRESH FRUIT PIE

Crust: 1 baked pie crust

Filling:
½ cup frozen orange juice concentrate
1 cup pineapple juice
3 Tbsp. agar-agar flakes
Maple syrup, fruit juice concentrate or other sweetener to taste, optional
6 cups assorted fresh fruit, cut bite-sized – frozen,
 unsweetened fruit can also be used (raspber-
 ries, blueberries, strawberries, peaches, apples,
 pears, pineapple, etc.)
Shredded, unsweetened coconut and fresh mint

In a small saucepan, heat the orange and pineapple juices. Add the starch or agar-agar and sweetener and stir until smooth and thick; remove from the heat and cool completely. Fold in the fresh fruit (drained) and turn into the baked crust. Garnish with coconut and fresh mint leaves. Serves 8.

PEACH COBBLER

6 cups sliced fresh peaches
½ cup peach nectar
1 cup oatmeal
⅓ cup ground pecans
¼ cup brown rice flour
1 tsp. ground cinnamon *and* a pinch of sea salt

¼ cup *each* maple syrup and raisins

Butter a pie plate; cover the bottom with the peaches and nectar. Combine the oatmeal, pecans, flour, cinnamon and syrup and mix well; sprinkle on the peaches, dot with butter, if desired, and bake until the peaches are soft. Top with ALMOND CREAM p. 94. Serves 8.

PECAN PIE

Crust: 1 granola pie crust, baked (see GRANOLA WITH DRIED FRUIT p. 71)

Filling:
¼ cup quick-cooking, granulated tapioca
1 cup apple juice
¼ cup *each* maple syrup and melted butter
1 tsp. vanilla extract
2 cups pecan halves or pieces

Place the tapioca and apple juice in a saucepan and cook on medium heat, stirring continuously, for about 5 minutes; the mixture should be fairly thick. Add the maple syrup and butter and stir until the butter is melted. Add the vanilla and pecans and mix until the pecans are well coated. Pour into the baked crust; bake at 350°F. for 20 minutes. Cool and serve with ALMOND or CASHEW CREAM pp. 94, 95. Serves 8.

PINEAPPLE-STRAWBERRY SHERBET

2 cups crushed pineapple, drained
6 oz. unsweetened pineapple juice concentrate
Sweetener to taste
1 pint of fresh strawberries, sliced
Fresh mint sprigs

Combine the pineapple, concentrate and sweetener and blend until smooth; pour into a shallow container and freeze semi-hard. Whisk until smooth and slushy; fold in the sliced strawberries and freeze until set. Garnish individual servings with fresh mint. Serves 4.

PINEAPPLE-TAPIOCA PUDDING OR PIE

2 cups unsweetened pineapple juice
½ cup quick-cooking, granulated tapioca
⅛ tsp. ground ginger
1 cup crushed pineapple, drained
3 Tbsp. maple syrup
Pinch of sea salt, optional
1 tsp. vanilla extract
1 cup CASHEW CREAM p. 95

In a saucepan, combine all the ingredients except the vanilla and cream; bring to a boil, reduce the heat and simmer for about 10 minutes, stirring continuously. Set aside to cool; then stir in the vanilla and cream.

For a Pudding: Refrigerate and serve in individual dishes with a garnish of fresh mint. Serves 6.

For a Pie: Bake a pie crust or a GRANOLA PIE CRUST p. 72; cool and fill with the pineapple-tapioca mixture. Chill well and garnish with fresh mint. Serves 8.

RICE PUDDING WITH (M)APPLE SYRUP

3 cups cooked BROWN RICE p. 92
½ cup seedless raisins
½ cup apple juice
2 cups NUT MILK p. 99
¼ cup NUT BUTTER p. 99
Finely grated rind of 1 lemon
½ tsp. ground nutmeg
2-3 Tbsp. sweetener (rice, barley or maple syrup)
1 tsp. molasses

2 eggs or equivalent egg replacer
½ tsp. vanilla extract
⅛ tsp. sea salt

Place the rice and raisins in a mixing bowl and set aside. Combine the remaining ingredients in a blender or food processor and blend well. Stir in the rice mixture and pour into an oiled baking dish. Bake at 325°F. for 1 hour or until slightly browned. Serve with (M) APPLE SYRUP p. 97. Serves 8.

STRAWBERRY PIE

Crust:
1 cup finely ground almonds
1 cup flour (unbleached, whole wheat, rice, soy)
2 Tbsp. butter or soy margarine, melted
2 Tbsp. maple syrup
2 Tbsp. cold water (more if needed)

Combine all the ingredients; mix well and press into an oiled pie plate. Bake at 400°F. for 10-15 minutes.

Filling:
1 pint strawberries, cut in half
¼ cup orange juice concentrate
½ cup apple juice concentrate
1 Tbsp. agar-agar

Topping:
ALMOND CREAM p. 94

Arrange the strawberry halves in the cooked pie crust. In a small saucepan, dissolve the agar-agar in the orange and apple juice concentrates and bring to a boil. Reduce the heat and simmer for 5 minutes, stirring constantly. Pour the glaze over the strawberries and chill until set, at least 1 hour. Top individual servings with ALMOND CREAM. Serves 8.

SWEET YAM TARTS

Crust: GRANOLA PIE CRUST p. 72, unbaked

Filling:
2 cups cooked yams
½ cup stock from potatoes (more to thin, if necessary)
1 egg or equivalent egg replacer
3 Tbsp. orange juice concentrate
1 tsp. ground cinnamon
½ tsp. ground ginger
½ tsp. ground cloves
½ tsp. ground allspice
1 tsp. vanilla extract
½ tsp. sea salt
½ cup raisins
ALMOND CREAM p. 94 or CASHEW CREAM p. 95
Shredded, unsweetened coconut

Mash the yams until smooth. Add the remaining ingredients except the cream and coconut and mix well. Spoon into the shells and bake at 350°F. for 30 minutes. Cool and serve. Top with ALMOND or CASHEW CREAM and shredded coconut. Makes 10 tarts.

Snacks

BANANA-NUT BREAD

4 cups flour (try 2 cups whole wheat, 2 cups unbleached
   or 2 cups rice flour, 2 cups unbleached wheat)
1 Tbsp. low-sodium baking powder
1 tsp. baking soda
½-1 tsp. sea salt
1 cup melted butter or soy margarine
½ cup apple juice concentrate
¼ cup maple syrup

2 eggs or equivalent egg replacer
5-6 overripe bananas, mashed
½ cup buttermilk
1 Tbsp. cider or rice vinegar
1 cup chopped walnuts
½ cup raisins or currants

Preheat the oven to 350°F. Sift the dry ingredients together; cut in the butter with a pastry blender. Combine the remaining ingredients; stir into the dry mix. Turn into 2 oiled loaf pans; bake for 45-50 minutes or until a toothpick comes out clean. Cool in the pans for 10 minutes; turn onto a rack. Makes 2 loaves.

CAROB CHIP-OATMEAL COOKIES

½ cup butter or soy margarine
¼ cup maple syrup
1 egg or equivalent egg replacer
½ tsp. vanilla extract
1¼ cups flour, sifted (try ¾ cup unbleached wheat, and
    ½ cup brown rice flour)
1 cup oatmeal
¼ tsp. sea salt
2 tsp. low-sodium baking powder
¼ cup carob chips
½ cup raisins
½ cup chopped nuts (pecans or walnuts)

Preheat the oven to 350°F. Melt the butter; add the maple syrup, egg or egg replacer and vanilla and beat until creamy. Sift together the flour, oatmeal, salt and baking powder; stir into the butter mixture. Then add the carob chips, raisins and nuts. Drop the batter by the tablespoonful onto an oiled cookie sheet, about ½-inch apart. Bake for 15 minutes or until golden brown. Makes about 1½ dozen.

FIG ROLL COOKIES

½ cup butter, melted
½ cup maple syrup
¼ cup buttermilk
1 tsp. vanilla extract
1½ cups sifted brown rice flour
1½ cups sifted unbleached wheat flour
½ tsp. salt
½ tsp. baking soda
2 Tbsp. egg replacer powder

In a large bowl, combine the wet ingredients. Add the flour and salt; knead into a ball and chill well. Preheat the oven to 350°F. Roll out the dough to a ¼-inch thickness and spread evenly with FIG WHIP (below). Roll into a long cylinder and cut into 1-inch sections; place on an oiled cookie sheet and bake until lightly browned, about 20 minutes. Makes 2 dozen.

FIG WHIP

1 cup thick coconut milk or CASHEW CREAM p. 95 or
    ALMOND CREAM p. 94
3 cups dried figs
1 Tbsp. ground sesame seeds
1 Tbsp. carob powder
2 Tbsp. raisins
1 tsp. fresh lemon juice, optional

Combine all the ingredients in a blender or food processor and blend until smooth; chill before serving. Spoon into fruit cups and garnish with a sprinkle of fresh coconut. Or use as a filling for FIG ROLL COOKIES (above). Serves 6-8.

HALVAH ON RICE CAKES

1 cup tahini (or sesame butter)
Maple syrup to taste

Stir the tahini until creamy (so the oil is well mixed with the pulp). Add the maple syrup slowly while stirring, until the mixture becomes thick and crumbly and as sweet as desired. Serve on rice cakes, crackers, biscuits, or a sweet bread (challah).

NUTTY COOKIES

2 cups *each* chopped cashews and pecans
2 cups oatmeal
6 Tbsp. carob powder
1 tsp. baking soda
½ cup butter or soy margarine, melted
1 egg or equivalent egg replacer
1 tsp. vanilla extract
½ cup maple syrup
1 Tbsp. cider or rice vinegar

Combine the dry ingredients in a large mixing bowl. In another bowl, combine the wet ingredients; mix well and stir into the dry mixture. Drop by the teaspoonful onto oiled cookie sheets; bake at 350°F. for 20 minutes. Makes about 3 dozen.

OATMEAL FRUIT BARS

½ cup butter or soy margarine, melted
¼ cup maple syrup
¼ cup apple juice concentrate
3 eggs or equivalent egg replacer
2 tsp. vanilla extract
2½ cups oatmeal
1 cup flour (unbleached, whole wheat, soy, rice, etc.)

3 tsp. low-sodium baking powder
½ tsp. sea salt
½ cup chopped nuts
½ cup raisins
1 cup combined, chopped dried dates, apricots, and
   apples

Preheat the oven to 325°F. Combine the wet ingredients
in a small bowl and set aside. In a large mixing bowl,
combine the remaining ingredients; add the wet mixture
and stir well. Spread in a rectangular baking pan and
bake for 30-35 minutes. Cool before cutting into squares.
Makes 3 dozen bars.

PEANUT BUTTER COOKIES

¼ cup butter or soy margarine, melted
¼-½ cup maple syrup
1 egg or equivalent egg replacer
1 cup peanut butter
1 tsp. vanilla extract
½ tsp. sea salt (needed only if unsalted peanut butter is
   used)
½ tsp. baking soda
1 Tbsp. vinegar
2 cups soy flour

Preheat the oven to 375°F. In a large mixing bowl,
combine the wet ingredients and beat until smooth. Sift
in the dry ingredients and mix well; taste and adjust for
desired sweetness. Roll the dough into 1-inch balls and
place on an oiled cookie sheet; flatten with a fork and
bake for about 15 minutes. Makes about 2 dozen cookies.